Working in Public Health

What can you contribute to improving and protecting the health of your community? Public health is becoming an increasingly central area of healthcare practice, and people working in public health come from a wide range of disciplines and backgrounds.

This practical and accessible book maps out the range of exciting and varied options open to people considering a career in public health, and provides helpful information on how to get there, either as a fully-fledged specialist or in an operational practitioner role. Designed especially for those wanting to learn about public heath, it looks at public health work in a range of settings, from health services to the commercial sector, and in a range of different roles, from health protection to public health intelligence.

Numerous personal accounts and case studies from highly experienced practitioners and specialists, as well as those new to their roles, illustrate what their roles involve and how they have had an impact on improving health and reducing inequality. This is the ideal book for anyone interested in putting public health at the centre of their working lives.

Fiona Sim is a part-time GP and clinical director of her local Clinical Commissioning Group. She is visiting professor at the University of Bedfordshire and honorary senior lecturer at the London School of Hygiene and Tropical Medicine. She is chair of the Royal Society for Public Health and was previously head of public health development at the English Department of Health.

Jenny Wright is a specialist in public health and fellow of the Faculty of Public Health. She has a long-standing interest in the multidisciplinary public health workforce and in developing public health capacity. She worked for the Department of Health on the 2008 public health competency framework and in 2010 led the team developing and launching the UK Public Health Careers website.

Working in Public Health

An introduction to careers in public health

Edited by Fiona Sim and Jenny Wright

Routledge
Taylor & Francis Group

LONDON AND NEW YORK

First published 2015
by Routledge
2 Park Square, Milton Park, Abingdon, Oxon OX14 4RN

and by Routledge
711 Third Avenue, New York, NY 10017

*Routledge is an imprint of the Taylor & Francis Group,
an informa business*

British Library Cataloguing-in-Publication Data
A catalogue record for this book is available from the British Library

Library of Congress Cataloging-in-Publication Data
Working in public health: an introduction to careers in public health/
edited by Fiona Sim and Jenny Wright.
   p.cm.
Includes bibliographical references.
I. Sim, Fiona, editor. II. Wright, Jenny, 1948– editor.
[DNLM: 1. Public Health – Great Britain. 2. Career Choice – Great
Britain. 3. Vocational Guidance – Great Britain. WA 21]
RA440.9
362.1023′41 – dc23
2014008314

ISBN: 978-0-415-62454-1 (hbk)
ISBN: 978-0-415-62455-8 (pbk)
ISBN: 978-0-203-10440-8 (ebk)

Typeset in Sabon
by Florence Production Ltd, Stoodleigh, Devon, UK

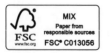

Printed and bound in Great Britain by
TJ International Ltd, Padstow, Cornwall

Contents

Foreword

I was delighted to be asked to write a short Foreword for this very timely book. There has never been a more interesting, or valuable, time to be a public health practitioner, with a myriad of opportunities to apply public health skills and knowledge in a wide variety of ways and across many sectors as this book so amply shows. Equally, we face many health challenges that we need public health practitioners to help us resolve. Since becoming Chief Executive of Public Health England, I have been impressed by the dedication, professionalism and 'can do' approach shown by so many people whom I have been able to meet across the country working in public health in different roles. I am sure you will find this book an inspiring as well as helpful read.

Duncan Selbie, Chief Executive, Public Health England

If someone had told me when I qualified in Medicine in 1979 that I would go on to be a public health physician, I doubt whether I would have believed them. To say that my exposure to what was then termed 'community medicine' had not inspired me was a substantial understatement. It simply didn't compare with the excitement of a Saturday night in a busy emergency department, admitting perhaps thirty patients, many requiring split-second decisions. Nor did it compare with the intellectual challenges of diagnosis, such as the young man I looked after with a pyrexia of unknown origin who turned out to have a renal cancer. So I set off on my chosen path, quickly passing my specialist exams to become a Member of the Royal College of Physicians, and started on the ladder towards a consultant post in internal medicine. And I enjoyed what I was doing. I began to accumulate the necessary skills, viewing patients through endoscopes passed from both ends, taking biopsies from livers and various parts of the gut, and becoming familiar with the rapidly changing nature of imaging (indeed, one of my earliest papers in the *British Medical Journal* described an innovative use of CT scanning). I particularly enjoyed talking to patients, unravelling their complex histories that would, hopefully, lead me to a diagnosis. But it was all too good to last. If I was to progress any further I would have to take time out for research, and in those days that meant spending time in a laboratory. So there I was, learning the basics of laboratory work, patiently waiting for my rabbits to produce antibodies to an especially obscure small peptide. Yet I was continuing my clinical work and it became increasingly clear that the work I was doing in the laboratory and that in the clinic or ward were almost totally divorced from one another. Crucially, as I became better at communicating with my patients I realised that, in very many cases, the solution to their problems was not within my gift. It seems remarkable but, in 1980s Belfast, I was seeing patients with scurvy and beri-beri. Moreover, I was realising how so many of my consultants, and certainly the best among them, were really public health specialists in disguise. They taught me the importance of understanding how different jobs in the linen industry influenced the risk of byssinosis, or Belfast's legacy of mesotheliomas from its shipbuilding industry. They introduced me to the basics of epidemiology, something that, remarkably, seemed to have been missing from my undergraduate lessons in community medicine. As the realisation dawned on me that a career in academic medicine would involve spending much time away from my patients and the stories they permitted me to learn from, I decided to make a move. I transferred to the training scheme for public health and, as they say, the rest is history.

I have been extremely fortunate. I have witnessed at first hand remarkable social, economic and political changes, including the collapse of communism in Europe, the breaking down of barriers in the European Union and the economic crisis created by greedy and incompetent financial institutions in 2008. I have played a small part in documenting the health effects of these changes, making what would otherwise have been invisible visible, and bearing witness to the suffering of the most vulnerable people in society. I have been privileged to work with many remarkable people, learning from their diverse experiences and disciplinary perspectives. And, as if to remind me that everything one learns is of some use, one of my recent papers even involved research using a different small peptide to understand the complex role of alcohol in heart disease in Russia. That laboratory work was not, as I feared at the time, entirely wasted. And I have been fortunate in being given a platform to speak truth to power, even though my words have not always attracted universal agreement, especially when taking on powerful vested interests such as the tobacco and alcohol industries.

Looking back, my career in public health has been more exciting than anything I could ever have imagined. Moreover, I would like to think that I have done some things that, ultimately, have helped to make the world a better place. But my story is one of many. Numerous others working as public health specialists and practitioners, in health services, central and local government, academia and civil society organisations can tell similar stories. And indeed, some of them now have done. In this excellent book, Fiona Sim and Jenny Wright have done us a great service by bringing together a diverse group of people who, using different skills, in different settings, to tackle different problems, have each contributed to a healthier, happier world. Together, they demonstrate the breadth of careers open to those with the wide range of skills required to practise public health and serve as an inspiration to others to follow in their footsteps. Those who do, when they reach the stage of looking back on their careers, will have the immense satisfaction of being able to say 'I made a difference'.

Martin McKee, Professor of European Public Health,
London School of Hygiene & Tropical Medicine

Part 1

Introduction
Fiona Sim and Jenny Wright

Introduction to the book and to public health

This book is an introduction to the world of public health careers. It will give you an understanding of what public health is, what issues public health practitioners are tackling and why they need tackling, a description of some of the roles and career paths that public health practitioners follow. Lastly, when you have been inspired by these roles, the book provides some signposts about where you can go to get more information.

The book is aimed at those who are starting on their career journeys and considering public health as an option, and who want more information on the range of opportunities. For those considering a move towards public health in mid-career, the book also has valuable information. It will be of interest to those who are teaching on public health courses as well as those providing careers advice to young and not-so-young people.

There is no internationally agreed definition of public health. The Alma Ata Declaration (WHO, 1978), Health for All (WHO, 1981) and the Ottawa Charter (WHO, 1986) contain the modern emphasis on securing wellbeing as well as absence of disease. Public health was defined for the UK in 1988 by the then Chief Medical Officer (CMO) in his *Report of the Committee of Inquiry into the Future Development of the Public Health Function* (Acheson, 1988) as 'the science and art of preventing disease, prolonging life and promoting health through the organised efforts of society'. This was subsequently added to by Derek Wanless in his second report on public health (2004) 'through the organised efforts and informed choices of society, organisations, public and private, communities and individuals'. With these definitions, therefore, public health has moved from being a relatively narrow discipline, based around a small professional workforce, to being the rightful consideration of the whole population.

What sets public health practitioners apart is their passion and desire to improve the health and wellbeing of the population and to reduce inequalities. They want to contribute to making the world a better place. They will use their skills in understanding the impact of disease and ill health on different communities to bring about change. They are also aware of the influence of broader social and environmental factors on health, as illustrated in the diagram below (Dahlgren and Whitehead, 1991).

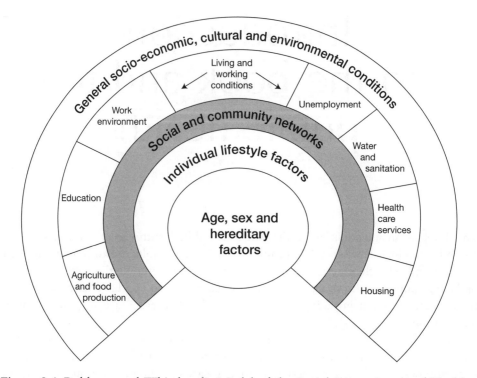

Figure 0.1 Dahlgren and Whitehead's Model of the Social Determinants of Health

Source: Dahlgren and Whitehead, 1991

The book is aimed at people considering or starting their public health careers from a UK base. We recognise that the arrangements for delivery of public health goals vary tremendously around the world, so that while many of the core competencies required will be the same, the organisation of services and jobs available may be very different from one country to another. Even within the UK there are country-specific differences. The book will not dwell upon these but we highlight where they are relevant to careers.

This book will show you the rich and varied opportunities for roles and careers in public health. Public health practitioners are found working in all walks of life – in the public, private and voluntary sectors. Many make their contribution in overseas work with developing countries.

What it means to work in public health

Working in public health means working to improve everyone's health, to prevent ill health and to make a real difference to people's lives. This is done in many different ways, so you will see that, unlike some other occupations, there is no single job or profession that sums up 'the public health practitioner'. What we tend to have in common, however, is a strong drive to improve the health and wellbeing of communities and an ability to have a long-term view, since many of the changes that are needed will take years or even decades to achieve.

Public health practitioners work as follows:

At local levels:

- with individuals and families;
- with and for local communities;
- with organisations that deliver services to individuals, families and communities (e.g. health services and local authorities, charities and independent organisations); and
- in teaching and research.

At regional or national levels:

- with organisations that plan services and develop policy (e.g. government departments, head offices for health services, social care organisations, charitable organisations, large companies).

At international and global levels:

- with organisations whose main focus is improving health outcomes in low- or middle-income settings (e.g. charitable organisations, United Nations organisations).

Changing public health issues

What have public health practitioners achieved for the population's health? The public health movement really began in the middle of the nineteenth century, in the face of diseases such as cholera and at a time of very high infant mortality. The focus of nineteenth- and early twentieth-century public health had been on understanding the causes of ill health and enabling major legislation to create:

- clean water and sanitation;
- safe food;
- safe working conditions; and
- fewer infectious diseases.

During the twentieth century, as the concepts of infection and contagious diseases became better understood, initial effort focused on reducing the threat of communicable and preventable diseases by measures such as immunisation programmes covering whole populations. In the 1940s, the main determinants of poor health were described in the Beveridge Report (Beveridge, 1942) as the 'Five Giants: Squalor, Ignorance, Want, Idleness, Disease'.

One major public health achievement in the UK at the end of the century was the introduction of seat-belt legislation to promote safety on roads. In the twenty-first century, the ban on smoking in public places has been an important step forward, in response to increasing understanding and political acceptance of the harmful effects on people's health from 'second-hand' tobacco smoke.

As a result of public health interventions, people are living longer and are healthier for longer, and there are fewer infant and child deaths, but there remain large inequalities in health between different groups within and between populations.

In the twenty-first century we have, however, a new set of challenges for the public health workforce in developed countries:

- management of chronic diseases and the impact of an ageing population;
- risks from new and emerging infectious diseases such as the severe acute respiratory syndrome (SARS) outbreak in 2002 and pandemics such as swine flu;
- climate change and its impact on health;
- widening inequalities in health, with poorer people being likely to have worse health and to live shorter lives than those who are more affluent;
- rapidly evolving lifestyle threats such as obesity and binge drinking of alcohol, as well as the continuing challenges posed by tobacco.

Global burden of disease

The average global life expectancy at birth is now 70 years, ranging from 60 years in low-income countries to 80 years in high-income countries (WHO, 2014). In many countries, more commonly low-income countries, there is no routine registration of diseases or of deaths and their cause, so that, while estimates are made, it is impossible to know accurately what diseases cause most ill health among populations worldwide, or which cause most deaths.

In the UK, and in many other high-income countries, information has been collected for decades that allows the health of the population to be tracked. Over time, the number of deaths from infectious diseases has declined – much of the improvement as a result of public health interventions such as clean water, better food hygiene and population-wide immunisation programmes – but deaths due to modern epidemics of heart disease, stroke and cancer have increased. Most of these modern scourges are linked with changes in society that have led to changes in diet, increased access to alcohol and tobacco, and lack of physical activity. Death is only one measure of health, of course, and the number of people who suffer long periods of ill health, particularly in older age, due to long-term conditions such as diabetes, circulatory diseases and dementia, are now of great importance to individuals and their families, and to the national economy, due to their major impact on demand for health and social care services. Unfortunately, the dream of the founding fathers of the NHS, who thought that the population would steadily become healthier and the need for healthcare would diminish, was somewhat flawed as many people live longer, but in poorer health. For public health practitioners the greatest challenge is to achieve healthy longevity – 'adding life to years as well as years to life' (Sim and McKee, 2011).

In response to these challenges, we need competent public health practitioners, working at all levels and in all settings. Whatever field of public health they work in, practitioners will need the following:

- awareness of differing health needs;
- knowledge of what influences our health and wellbeing;
- understanding of how to prevent ill health and promote health.

They will need skills in:

- communicating effectively;
- working successfully in collaboration with others, to influence and negotiate;
- analysing and interpreting information on people and health;
- reviewing literature on what makes a difference.

Introducing the public health workforce

The workforce is *multidisciplinary*, which means that public health practitioners come from a very wide range of initial disciplines and backgrounds. This can include medicine, nursing and other health professions, teaching, management, pharmacy, science, geography, mathematics, nutrition and the civil service. Increasingly, recruits to the public health workforce are from recent college and university graduates from a very wide range of subjects.

Public health practitioners operate at all levels, from those just entering the workforce at the very start of their careers, to senior strategic leaders and eminent professors. Practitioners work in all areas of the health service (primary care, hospitals, health boards and commissioning units), universities, local government and civil service in the public sector and also in the independent and voluntary sectors.

Public health practitioners work mainly in one of several broad fields or domains of practice. Understanding these will help to explain more simply how a career in public health may be developed, although in practice many people work across two or three or more of the domains at some time during their career.

1 Improving health

Health improvement practitioners work actively to improve people's health and wellbeing and work towards preventing disease and ill health. This can involve working with individuals to give advice about healthy changes to their lifestyle (such as healthy eating or regular exercise) or with communities and the media to promote health campaigns (such as healthy eating or safer sex), commissioning of health improvement programmes or to advocate or help to plan changes to public policy.

Examples of roles in the workplace include smoking cessation advisers, community development officers, health promotion specialists and population screening programme managers.

Those considering health improvement careers may have enjoyed learning about education, sociology, psychology, marketing, communications and anthropology.

2 Protecting health

Health protection practitioners promote safety in the workplace (such as fire safety or the safe handling of goods) or the safety of the wider population (such as ensuring the safety of food, or protecting people from infectious diseases and environmental hazards, such as noise, chemicals or radiation).

Examples of roles in the workforce include environmental health officers, infection control nurses, consultants in communicable disease control and emergency planning officers.

Those considering health protection careers may have enjoyed learning about biology, chemistry, epidemiology, environmental health, infectious diseases, laboratory techniques, health screening, emergency response and engineering.

3 Maintaining and raising standards of health and social care

Healthcare public health practitioners are interested in raising the standard of services provided to the public to help improve their health, and in making sure that public health is a safe and effective service. This might include developing specifications and setting priorities for others to provide particular services, as well as commissioning services, researching and advising on the evidence base for the effectiveness of services.

Examples of roles in the workplace include clinical governance officers and clinical effectiveness managers.

Those considering healthcare public health careers may have enjoyed learning about business, economics, public policy, project management, clinical governance, and service audit and quality.

4 Working with information (health intelligence)

Health intelligence practitioners collect, analyse, interpret and communicate information about health. This information can be about the general health and wellbeing of the whole population, or about the health risks and health needs of a particular social group (such as an age group or an ethnic group).

Examples of roles in the workplace include cancer intelligence officers and information analysts in public health teams and units.

Those considering health intelligence careers may have enjoyed learning about mathematics, statistics, epidemiology, basic sciences, computer sciences and database management.

5 Working in academic public health (teaching and researching)

Academic public health practitioners are interested in investigating public health issues or teaching about public health. This can involve teaching about public health in a university or college, or setting up research projects to investigate specific public health issues (such as obesity, hospital cleanliness, climate change) and publishing the results.

Examples of roles in the workplace include public health research officers and lecturers in public health.

Those considering academic public health careers may have enjoyed learning about education, research methods, epidemiology, evidence-based policy and practice, and monitoring and evaluation.

6 Leading strategic planning, management and policy development

Strategic planning public health practitioners are interested in leading work to improve the health and wellbeing of the population, in developing initial policy, the strategies to put the plans into action, strategic commissioning of appropriate services, overseeing implementation, and in measuring the impact that policies and strategies have on the quality of health and wellbeing services, and the outcomes for individuals and communities.

Examples of roles in the workplace include policy officers, consultants in public health and directors of public health.

Those considering careers in policy and strategic leadership may have enjoyed learning about public policy, health services management and health scrutiny.

How we categorise the public health workforce

There is no rigid definition of who is in the public health workforce. Often, the words 'public health' do not feature in job titles. The following three categories were developed in 2001 and best describe the composition of the public health workforce (Donaldson, 2001).

Wider workforce

This group includes those who have a role in health improvement, protecting health and reducing inequalities but who would not necessarily regard themselves as part of the public health/health and wellbeing workforce.

This is the largest group in the workforce and includes the front-line health service and local government workforces such as care assistants, teachers and nurses who, through their interactions with patients or members of the public, can provide advice on lifestyle or signpost where people who need more information can go.

Practitioners

People working in this group spend a major part or all of their time in public health practice. They work in multiprofessional teams and include people who work with groups and communities as well as with individuals. They have knowledge and in-depth skills for their particular areas of practice.

This is the second largest group and includes the workforce responsible for much of the delivery of public health programmes such as health promotion, health visiting and school nursing, public health nutrition, information on health status and environmental health. Some, but not all, groups in the public health practitioner workforce have formal professional qualifications and are regulated through specific organisations.

Public health specialists

This group includes consultants and specialists who work at strategic or senior management level, or at a senior level of scientific expertise such as in public health statistics. At this level, an ability to manage change, lead public health programmes and work across organisational boundaries is crucial, as are technical skills in epidemiology, health promotion or healthcare evaluation.

This is the smallest group in the workforce and anyone working at this level is qualified in public health at specialist level and usually registered formally with one of the three bodies for specialist regulation.

This book concentrates mainly on people who work in public health at either operational or strategic levels – that is, practitioners and specialists. Do remember, however, as illustrated by some of the career stories in this book, that often people who find themselves drawn to being in either of these categories in mid-career have themselves come from the wider public health workforce.

Broad outline of careers in public health

Careers in public health are rewarding, challenging and also hugely varied. For some practitioners, qualification routes are straightforward, such as environmental health where there are specific courses, qualifications and regulation (by the Chartered Institute of Environmental Health for England, Wales and Northern Ireland, and by The Royal Environmental Health Institute of Scotland). Public health nurses have all undertaken specific courses and are regulated by the Nursing and Midwifery Council.

Other roles, such as health promotion officers and health intelligence officers, currently do not have specific, regulated, national standards that practitioners are required to meet, but many will have undertaken a relevant undergraduate and often a postgraduate course, usually at Master's level. Since April 2011, through several local pilot schemes, some public health practitioners have elected to meet voluntary standards and register formally as public health practitioners with the UK Public Health Register.

For those wishing to qualify as a specialist and achieve the status of consultant in public health, the principal route is to apply for a place on the specialist training scheme, which has an annual national recruitment round and is open to applicants from any background who meet the entry criteria. Training normally takes five years and includes passing the Faculty of Public Health examinations and meeting all their competence requirements. Those signed off as competent are then eligible for specialist registration with, for doctors, the General Medical Council (GMC) and the UK Public Health Register (all other disciplines). Public health dentists have a separate, but equivalent, specialist training scheme in dental public health and are regulated by the General Dental Council (GDC).

Regulation at either specialist or practitioner level is for the protection of the public and recognition that individuals have met professional standards. Those registered must keep their skills and knowledge up to date (continuing professional development (CPD)) and demonstrate that they have maintained competence by periodically undergoing revalidation, a recently introduced system for ensuring up-to-date knowledge and skills in the regulated workforce.

Most public health careers are flexible and it is rare for practitioners to spend their whole career in one organisation. Practitioners working in public health may move employer and type of employment. A health visitor, for example, may become interested in undertaking formal training to become a public health consultant, or a screening officer may become interested in health intelligence and undertake further study in health informatics and move to a health intelligence post. The career stories in this book will illustrate the variety of paths taken by public health practitioners.

Public health competence

In recent years in the UK, public health competence has been divided by convention into four core areas, which anyone working in the public health field will normally need to have skills in, and five defined areas relating to specific skills needed for different areas of practice. At the most senior (consultant) level, all practitioners are required to show they are competent across all nine areas.

Core competence areas:

- surveillance and assessment;
- assessing the evidence;
- policy and strategy; and
- leadership and collaborative working.

Competences in defined areas of practice:

- health improvement;
- health protection;

- public health intelligence;
- academic public health; and
- health and social care quality.

There is a competency framework that sets out in more detail these competencies and how they apply to nine different career levels – that is, they will relate to all three categories of the public health workforce (UK Public Health Skills and Career Framework, Skills for Health,[1] 2008). On the UK Public Health Careers website, PHORCaST[2] (www.phorcast.org.uk) the competency framework is set out in full. It offers a quick checklist for site visitors to be able to assess for themselves what competencies they have at different levels in the workforce and what competencies they might need for specific roles.

Current organisation of public health workforces in the four UK countries

England, with a population (Office of National Statistics Census, 2011) of 53 million, is by far the largest of the four UK countries. Scotland, at the same time, had a population of 5.3 million, Wales 3.1 million and Northern Ireland 1.8 million.

Since the 1990s, the health systems in the four countries have become increasingly divergent as responsibility for the organisation of health and social care has been within the remits of devolved administrations. For example, England is now the only one of the four countries to retain a full internal market with purchaser–provider[3] split in healthcare. This has had an impact on both the configuration and what is required of the public health workforce. Also in England only, most of the local public health workforce has been transferred out of the NHS to work within local government since April 2013.

England: new public health system from April 2013

The new system is based on the coalition government's White Paper *(Healthy Lives, Healthy People: Our Strategy for Public Health in England)*, issued by the Department of Health on 30 November 2010 and set in statute by the Health and Social Care Act 2012. This set up two principal arrangements for the future employment of the public health workforce – as part of either a new national public health agency, Public Health England (PHE), or within (upper tier[4]) local government. Those moving to PHE were primarily practitioners working in the fields of health protection or health intelligence, but also include some health improvement practitioners and those working on specialised services commissioning as well as the commissioning of screening programmes. Those moving into local government were primarily practitioners working in the field of health improvement. Practitioners working in the field of healthcare moved either to PHE or local government, with few remaining in the NHS.

The new agency is operating as a single organisation working on a distributed model with regional teams, centres, and knowledge and intelligence teams. Some staff are outposted to Area Teams within NHS England to support specific commissioning functions.

The Health and Social Care Act 2012 gave new statutory responsibilities for public health to local authorities. To carry out these responsibilities councils have funding to commission public health programmes such as sexual health, smoking cessation and other specific public health teams, led by a Director of Public Health (joint appointment between the local authority and Secretary of State). These teams will also provide public health advice to local health service commissioners.

Wales

The Welsh Assembly Government is responsible for the funding and oversight of NHS Wales, and other health and social care-related bodies.

The public health workforce for Wales is employed by Public Health Wales, an NHS Trust, which delivers specialist public health services to the Welsh Assembly Government as well as support to the local health boards through Directors of Public Health and their teams. The Wales model contrasts with the new Public Health England model in that the whole of the specialist and practitioner public health workforce is employed within Public Health Wales and staff operate on a matrix model, balancing countrywide responsibilities with local support.

Scotland

The Scottish Government Department for Health and Wellbeing is responsible for NHS Scotland, and for formulating and implementing health and community care policy.

NHS Scotland comprises fourteen NHS Boards responsible for the planning and delivery of all health services in their own area. In addition, there are eight Special Health Boards in Scotland, which include NHS Health Scotland (Scotland's main health improvement agency) and NHS Education for Scotland (NES). The public health workforce is primarily employed within one of these boards or agencies.

The Scottish Health Boards all have large public health departments, which employ (mainly medical) consultants and multidisciplinary teams that deliver health improvement, health intelligence, advice on healthcare and health protection services. There is a public health network spanning all Health Boards.

Northern Ireland

The Department of Health, Social Services and Public Safety for Northern Ireland (DHSSPS) is one of eleven Northern Ireland Government Departments created in 1999 as part of the Northern Ireland Executive. The DHSSPS carries overall responsibility to the Northern Ireland Assembly for the provision of health and social care services in Northern Ireland. Northern Ireland has had integrated health and social services since 1975.

Working under the DHSSPS, the Health and Social Care Board (HSCB) is responsible for commissioning services, managing resources allocated by the DHSSPS and performance improvement.

A Northern Ireland-wide Public Health Agency was created in April 2009, incorporating all public health practitioners.

Structure of this book

Because of the rich variety of public health careers, one book on its own cannot cover all possible roles and opportunities. Rather, what the contributors and editors have done is to use personal accounts from practitioners and specialists, at different stages in their careers, to inspire and illustrate as well as provide practical information. Each contributor covers the overall function or setting, the ways it can contribute to improving the health of the population and reducing inequalities, indication of specific roles in the setting or function, examples of where public health practitioners and specialists have made a difference, what it is like to work in different settings or functions – the challenges and rewards – career opportunities in this field and how to get going if you are interested in this kind of career. Some accounts are very personal and provide the contributor's own public health career journey. Some relate more to the specific organisation in which they work. Views are the contributors' own. Where appropriate, contributors have listed specific resources for interested readers to explore further.

Accounts cover the main areas of public health practice as well as the main settings in which public health practitioners work, give practical advice on what to expect from a range of roles and how to attain them. For anyone wishing to have more detail on specific careers, qualifications and courses, or to read other career stories, the UK Public Health Careers website (www.phorcast.org.uk) will provide further information.

Acknowledgements

This book would not have been possible without the willingness of all the contributors to share their insights, knowledge and career stories. We are indebted to them all and delighted to bring this composite story to a wide readership, some of whom we know will be inspired as a result to strive towards establishing their own successful career as a public health practitioner. We are also grateful to many other people who have shown great enthusiasm for this book, encouraged us and told us how timely it is, shared their ideas freely and made suggestions for contributors for the book.

Notes

1 Sector Skills Council for Health.
2 We, the editors, have received authoritative advice (April 2014) that the name PHORCaST will not be 'lost' until around the end of 2014, when this much-valued resource will become one section of what we are advised is likely to be called a national 'health careers' website with links through to the public health pages.
3 Internal market with commissioners of healthcare in separate organisations from those providing healthcare. Introduced in England in 2002.
4 County councils, unitary authorities or metropolitan boroughs.

References

Acheson, D. Report of the Committee of Inquiry into the Future Development of the Public Health Function, Cmd 289, London, HMSO, 1988.

Beveridge, W. (Chair) Social Insurance and Allied Services (SIAS), Cmd 6404, London, HMSO, 1942.

Dahlgren, G. and Whitehead, M. Policies and Strategies to Promote Social Equity in Health. Stockholm, Institute for Future Studies, 1991.

Donaldson, L. Report of the Chief Medical Officer's Project to Strengthen the Public Health Function in England, London, Department of Health, 2001.

Department of Health, Healthy People, Healthy Lives: Our Strategy for Public Health in England, Cm 7985, London, Department of Health, 2010. Available online at: www.gov.uk/government/uploads/system/uploads/attachment_data/file/216096/dh_127424.pdf. Accessed 22 June 2014.

Sim, F. and McKee, M. (eds) *Issues in Public Health*, 2nd edn, Maidenhead, Open University Press, 2011.

Skills for Health, *UK Public Health Skills and Career Framework*, April 2008. Available online at: www.skillsforhealth.org.uk/search/public%20health/?ordering=newest&search phrase=all. Accessed 10 November 2013.

UK Public Health Careers website: www.phorcast.org.uk.

Wanless, D. Securing Good Health for the Whole Population, Final Report, London, HMSO, 25 February 2004.

World Health Organization (WHO) Primary Health Care: Report of the International Conference on Primary Health Care, Alma-Ata, USSR, 6–12 September 1978, Geneva, WHO, 1978.

World Health Organization (WHO) Global Strategy for Health for All by the Year 2000, Geneva, WHO, 1981.

World Health Organization (WHO) Ottawa Charter for Health Promotion, First International Conference on Health Promotion, Geneva, WHO, October, 1986.

World Health Organization (WHO) Global Burden of Disease Project. Available online at: www.who.int/healthinfo/global_burden_disease/en. Accessed 4 January 2014.

Part 2

Public health functions
Fiona Sim and Jenny Wright

This part illustrates the diversity of work in public health. It includes accounts from a range of public health practitioners who describe their experience delivering different contemporary public health functions. It is important to remember that for each of these functions, the practitioner may be able to work in a variety of settings. The functions described in this part are:

- health improvement/health promotion.
- health intelligence/health informatics.
- healthcare/health service public health.
- health protection (including control of communicable diseases).
- academic public health (including public health research and public health teaching); and
- global health.

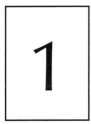

1

Health improvement

Richard Parish; Em Rahman

Introduction to this function

Health improvement practitioners work actively to improve people's health and wellbeing. This can involve working with individuals to give advice about healthy changes to their lifestyle (such as healthy eating or regular exercise) or with communities and the media to promote health campaigns (such as stopping smoking or having safer sex) or to advocate changes to public policy. Examples of roles in the workforce are smoking cessation advisers, community development officers and health promotion specialists.

EXAMPLES OF PUBLIC HEALTH PRACTITIONER ROLES FOR THIS FUNCTION

The contributions cover two very different perspectives, from influencing policy at the national level to how to change individual lifestyle behaviour as part of the front-line workforce.

Richard Parish, former Chief Executive, Royal Society for Public Health

A life in health promotion: what is health promotion?

Health promotion, often referred to as health improvement, is one of the major strands of contemporary public health. Together with health protection, it forms one of the two fundamental pillars in a continuum of activities designed to protect and promote population health and wellbeing. The third public health dimension ensures that health and social care and other services are planned and delivered to suit the health needs of specific communities.

Health can be viewed as a continuum. At one end of the spectrum we have severe illness or avoidable disability. Health protection aims to avoid both individuals and whole populations sliding towards poorer health, often as a result of communicable disease, environmental degradation or major disasters. By contrast, health promotion focuses on moving people towards their potential for optimum health. They may not currently be ill, but are nevertheless some distance from enjoying the best possible level of health.

$$\text{Severe ill health} \xleftarrow{\text{Health protection}} \text{X} \xrightarrow{\text{Health promotion}} \text{Optimum health}$$
$$\text{Average health}$$

At its simplest, health protection is concerned with reducing the risk of our health status shifting to the left, while health promotion is all about moving it to the right. They are complementary strategies.

Health is determined by a complexity of interrelated factors. Our biological make-up is, of course, fixed genetically, but whether or not individual genes express themselves, and to what extent, may well be determined by a wide variety of environmental and social influences. In any event, even if we have a genetic predisposition to a particular ill-heath outcome – say, heart disease – there is much we can do to ameliorate the risk and, in so doing, enhance our capacity for everyday living. Health promotion is about helping people achieve their potential for health and wellbeing.

Many of the influences on health are beyond the capacity of any individual to change. We are all products of the circumstances in which we grow and live. Our family situation, societal values, behavioural norms, economic circumstances and physical environment all determine our health prospects. Of course, the healthcare system also plays an important part, but it is these wider determinants of health that largely influence our health outcomes. The food we eat, the mass media to which we are exposed, the way our roads and cities are designed, the laws we pass, the goods we tax, all impact on our health-related behaviour. We are not creatures of free will in the way that most of us would like to believe, but products of the way our societies are organised and the prevailing social norms and cultural values.

Skills needed

Health promotion practitioners are concerned with all these fundamental influences on health. The discipline requires an understanding of social psychology, human biology, the processes of policy formulation, media planning, ecology and environmental design, and organisational management. Most of all, it demands an ability to make connections between a multitude of overlapping and interlocking factors – to see the whole rather than just the sum of the parts. Health promotion does not just focus on the individual, but sees the person in the context of their family, community and wider society.

For example, it is sometimes said that 'we are what we eat' and, to some extent, this is a truism. But how much control as individuals do we really have over our diet? The human food chain is influenced at every stage from primary agricultural production through to the consumer information available at the time we exercise a food-related choice. Never mind the current debate about genetically modified foods, decades (sometimes centuries) of selective breeding have created the animals and plants we eat. Many of them are substantially altered from their original undomesticated or unmodified forebears. Add to this the additional production stages before reaching our mouths involving food processing, manufacturing, marketing and product labelling, and we have a whole variety of decisions taken for a multitude of reasons that have nothing to do with health or decent nutrition. The financial considerations involved in agriculture and production, how best to recycle what otherwise might be viewed as waste products (e.g. hidden fat) and the cost-related specifications laid down by major retailers, all determine the choices available to us when we go to the supermarket or select from the menu in our local take-away. Our ability to exercise true choice is limited; it requires the collective act of society to change these fundamental determinants of health. *Enter the health promotion practitioner.*

Our potential for health is clearly driven by a number of influences and it is unlikely that any one individual will have all the knowledge and skills required for effective health promotion. It is by definition a team effort. Those entering the field come from a variety of 'feeder' disciplines – the social and biological sciences, education, the healthcare professions, and human geography or environmental science, to name but a few. It is not unknown for people to be recruited from other disciplines as well, such as the arts, linguistics, the physical sciences or history. Indeed, historians can provide a unique perspective, given the importance that population health has played in human, social and scientific development over the years. Whatever the starting point, most health promotion practitioners undertake a Master's-level qualification in either public health or, more specifically, health promotion either directly after their first degree or within a short period following recruitment into a health improvement role. It is increasingly common for people to study part-time alongside their day job.

My career journey

My own journey might be regarded as slightly unconventional. I started my career with a degree in the biological sciences. My particular interests were ecology, social biology and the impact of evolutionary pressures at a population level. Clearly, the seeds for a career in health promotion and public health were being sown at an early stage, although I did not recognise it at the time. Indeed, I was wholly unaware that the NHS employed people to work in health promotion (or health education as it was known at the time).

My Bachelor's degree in Biology was followed by a teaching certificate, specialising in adult education. Although perhaps less challenging than now, as there were far fewer university graduates, competition for graduate jobs in the mid-1970s was nevertheless considerable. Initially, I applied for and was offered a fixed term NHS administrative position in child health services. This opened my eyes to a wide range of health-related occupations and, perhaps more importantly, improved my under-standing of health and the influences on it. I moved to a more senior, permanent position in primary care and at the same time taught human biology in the evenings at the local college of further education. My position in the NHS provided access to the vast array of employment opportunities advertised in the journals, a veritable smorgasbord of careers and occupations. Among these I discovered the 'Health Education Officer', described in more recent decades as 'health promotion', 'health development' or 'health improvement'. Further investigation of the role fuelled my interest and I applied for a trainee position in the West Midlands.

At the time, most recruits came from community nursing, often health visiting. It was still unusual for graduates to be appointed, although the tide was certainly turning. I had the good fortune to be appointed from a large field, including at least two on the shortlist with doctorates. This was almost unheard of at the time, although it reflected the increasing labour market pressures of the mid to late 1970s.

Whatever the reasons for my appointment, I found myself working for a delightful, energetic and insightful Area Health Education Officer, who headed up her service within the local health authority. Although from a more traditional health-visiting background, she had a broad understanding of the wider societal influences upon health. A joy to work with, she acted as coach and mentor during my inauguration into the world of health promotion and public health. I spent a few months in my trainee role and was then seconded for an academic year to study for the Postgraduate Diploma (now M.Sc.) in Health Education at London South Bank University. At the time, this was one of only two higher education institutions offering the qualification, the other being Leeds Metropolitan University. A third institution, Bristol Polytechnic (now the University of the West of England) was added not long after. These days, some fifty or so UK universities offer similar programmes of study. I returned to the West Midlands following successful completion of the South Bank course.

Upon returning to Dudley Area Health Authority, I was soon to learn that the local population suffered a disproportionately high incidence of perinatal mortality (stillbirths and deaths in the first week after birth). My boss encouraged me to take this on as a special responsibility and I started to investigate the possible causes of Dudley's aberrant perinatal statistics, which, for the families involved, represented a personal tragedy. Working with the local community midwives and in discussion with new mothers in the areas of major population growth, we concluded that a range of factors was contributing to the high perinatal mortality. The assumption in the upper echelons of the local NHS community health services was that a more comprehensive antenatal educational programme was needed to teach expectant mothers how best to look after their health and that of their baby during the various stages of pregnancy. Not only was this patronising and condescending, it turned out to be a wholly inaccurate diagnosis of the problem. Appropriate and timely access to antenatal health services, the knowledge and attitudes of the healthcare practitioners themselves, and local transport arrangements were the root causes of the high perinatal mortality in this part of the Midlands. Remedial action was taken in all these areas, resulting in noticeable improvements in the perinatal statistics. I would contend that this was an early example of action on the wider determinants of health, which are largely beyond the influence of individuals and their families. This was a conceptual leap of understanding on my part, one that influenced my approach to public health throughout the rest of my career. It also taught me the value of skills, such as negotiation tactics and media management, that were not apparent in the postgraduate curricula at that time, although they are now.

The work in Dudley led to my first publication, an article in the *Health Services Journal*, which laid out a model for planning community-based health promotion programmes. This formative time in Dudley, supported by a visionary boss, provided the springboard for my subsequent career and taught me the value of 'on the job' experience as well as academic qualifications. It is in the laboratory of real life that we really hone our skills, as opposed to building our knowledge base, and we still have much more to do in establishing a meaningful coaching and mentoring scheme that supports practitioners through the different phases of their career development.

In 1980, after a much shorter period rising through the ranks than would now normally be the case, I was appointed as Area Health Promotion Officer for Stockport Health Authority, a somewhat meteoric rise for which I was less well equipped than I thought! At the time of my appointment, Stockport had a young and dynamic Area Medical Officer (the equivalent now is Director of Public Health) and it was at his instigation that I was appointed. Stockport did not have its own health promotion service at the time, not even the accommodation to house one, and I duly set about establishing a new department with all the naivety and inexperience, but enthusiasm, of relative youth. The Stockport Health Promotion Service was soon established. We were among the very first, sometimes the first, to establish community-wide plans on such issues as smoking, diet and nutrition, and alcohol. We set up a unique and successful scheme to redistribute safety equipment to support disadvantaged households and developed the concept of a Community Health Centre, which bore little resemblance to the primary care clinics in evidence today.

To the best of my knowledge, Stockport was the first health authority to have a published five-year strategy for health improvement. Unlike plans elsewhere, Stockport's approach was based on the settings where people lived out their daily lives – the workplace, schools and neighbourhoods. The move away from delivering disease-based prevention programmes, such as cancer and cardio-vascular disease, to an integrated settings approach was controversial at the time and severely criticised in some quarters. Within three years, however, Stockport was designated as the NHS Health Promotion Demonstration Centre, an accolade guaranteed to upset colleagues elsewhere, and I was appointed by the Secretary of State for Health to serve on the Board of the Health Education Council, the national body for England, Wales and Northern Ireland. This was my introduction to the politics of health, writ large!

The importance of understanding health promotion at the local, regional and national levels was becoming apparent. They are all interlinked, each providing a context for what is or is not possible at other levels of community organisation. Continuing this theme, my next appointment took me to Wales as Director of Programmes for the world's largest heart health initiative, 'Heartbeat Wales'. The sheer scale of this project, working with a population of almost three million, provided a real opportunity to tackle the whole range of health determinants in an integrated fashion. Service reconfiguration, innovative use of the mass media and influencing the human food supply chain all become possible with large-scale initiatives. It was as part of the Heartbeat Wales programme that the 'Exercise on Prescription' idea was born. After three years, Heartbeat Wales was being described by the Director General of the World Health Organization as the world's most significant health promotion programme.

Heartbeat Wales created many new learning opportunities, including the freedom to experiment and evaluate. In my subsequent management roles I have always tried to establish a similar culture. People and organisations grow when their creativity is allowed to flourish, while evaluation enables us to learn what works and to share the evidence widely.

Heartbeat Wales helped to reinforce the contribution made by all economic sectors to health and wellbeing. Gone were the days when it was all about the public sector. Third sector bodies both represent and energise civic society, providing a focal point for the organised actions of large numbers of people, many of them unpaid volunteers. As for the private sector, commercial organisations supply so many of the goods and services that determine our health. I was able to learn about these other sectors through my direct engagement with them and, as a consequence, ended up as a member of the Meat and Livestock Commission for Wales.

Stockport had given me the opportunity to meet with colleagues from the world-famous Finnish heart disease prevention programme in North Karelia. Despite their pre-eminent reputation in heart health promotion, they were extremely interested in the innovative work underway in the Stockport area. The partnership with Finland was the start of a career-long involvement in international health. The move to Wales provided further opportunities for international exchange and in 1986 my colleagues and I had the opportunity to help develop the Ottawa Charter for Health Promotion (First International Conference on Health Promotion, 1986). This has continued to provide the conceptual framework for health promotion right up to the present day.

Throughout my time at Stockport and in Wales, I continued my academic and professional development. I completed the process for registration as a chartered biologist, registered for the distance learning Certificate in Health Economics at Aberdeen University and became a member of both the Institute of Health Services Management and the Royal Society for Public Health. A research degree followed in the early nineties. Health promotion and public health embrace virtually every discipline imaginable, and one of the great personal benefits of a career in this field is that it is a lifelong learning journey. One can never become bored or master every facet and nuance of the work.

My next career move, just on the cusp of 1989 becoming 1990, took me beyond public health. I was appointed Chief Executive of the first fully multidisciplinary NHS higher education college, covering North Lincolnshire and East Yorkshire. This was a major challenge for me, both as an educational leader and as an NHS Chief Executive. The new college rapidly took on a national role and I realised with hindsight just how transferable the skills are that we acquire in health promotion. Problem analysis and definition, whole system planning, organisational change, people management, and monitoring and evaluation – they are the bedrock for managing complex organisations, whatever the sector. Some five years later the decision was taken nationally to merge all the NHS colleges with universities and I moved to Sheffield

Hallam University as Director of the School of Health and Community Studies, then two years later to a similar appointment at the University of York. Although these were primarily management roles, I was able to continue to make a contribution to research and teaching in public health throughout my time in higher education.

In 1999 I moved to become Chief Executive of the Health Education Authority, shortly to become the Health Development Agency (HDA) for England. In 2003, I left to undertake international consultancy work, predominantly for the World Health Organization (WHO). The HDA's functions transferred to the National Institute for Health and Care Excellence (NICE) in 2005.

My work for the WHO during the early part of the first decade of the new millennium provided some wonderful challenges. Following the 9/11 attacks on New York and Washington, I was asked by the European Director for the WHO to coordinate and produce the health plan for Europe in the event of a biological, chemical or radiation attack. The report was approved unanimously by the fifty-two countries of the European region. This work was new to me, although once again I discovered the value of my health promotion transferable skill set. An appointment to lead the 2005 European Health Report followed and, almost in parallel, to research and draft the European Strategy for Child and Adolescent Health and Development.

In 2005 it was time to rejoin the ranks of the employed, as opposed to the rather more precarious existence as a freelancing consultant: I was appointed as CEO to the Royal Society of Health (RSH) in June 2005. In that role, supported by trustees of both organisations, I led the merger of the RSH with another public health charity, the Royal Institute of Public Health, to become CEO of the new Royal Society for Public Health, in 2008. Through the endeavours of the staff, members and trustees, this has now achieved national acclaim for much of its work.

Crucially, we established a proper relationship between governance and the everyday management of the organisation. This allowed staff the freedom to use their knowledge and skills, while ensuring robust accountability. For my part, I was able to deploy all the experience and skills I had acquired in earlier incarnations, including the importance of a commercial approach to managing finance. In the charitable ('third') sector, one views income and expenditure through a different lens when every penny has to be earned in a market-orientated world and where success is determined primarily by the price and quality of the products and services on offer.

Having worked a seven-day week for much of my professional life, I stepped down from the RSPH at the end of June 2013 in order to lead a more balanced existence. I am not ready to retire and, to my good fortune, I have been asked to undertake a number of interesting part-time or non-executive roles.

Reflections on my career

So what have I learned as I move towards the sunset years of my career in health promotion and public health? To start with, the skills we acquire in health promotion with respect to organisational and individual behaviour change, including advocacy, are transferable to a wide variety of circumstances and situations. Second, the knowledge we have in planning, management and evaluation also has widespread application, but knowledge without employment-based competencies diminishes our ability to be effective. Even if we have the knowledge and skills for the job, health promotion demands ongoing tenacity, often in the face of adversity and political resistance. Third, health promotion at its core unifies thinking and experience from many disciplines and sectors. As such, it is a never-ending learning experience, but this is also its joy and reward.

Finally, the race for better health is an unending marathon. There will always be a need for the right people with the right skills, energy and commitment, if we are ever going to come close to achieving our potential for health and wellbeing. And in building our human capital we are more likely to create content, equitable and economically viable societies in the process.

Em Rahman, Public Health Workforce Development, Wessex Deanery

Health trainers, a public health workforce

The following quotation describes a very hands-on role in health promotion, as a health trainer at a local operational level.

> Health Trainers are a key tool to promote healthier lifestyles and reduce health inequalities. They reach out to people who are in circumstances that put them at a greater risk of poor health and work with them to assess their health and lifestyle risks, helping them to build their motivation to change. Health Trainers have facilitated behaviour change and provided advice, motivation and practical support to individuals in their local communities since 2006.
>
> (Marmot, 2009)

The Health Trainer programme

Health trainers were first identified in 2004 in the government's Public Health White Paper, *Choosing Health: Making Healthier Choices Easier* (Department of Health, 2004), which set out plans to provide more of the opportunities, support and information that the public want in order to enable them to make healthier and more informed choices regarding their health. The White Paper gave a commitment that from 2006 NHS health trainers would be developed to provide advice, motivation and practical support to individuals in their local communities.

The key underpinning philosophy of the Health Trainer Programme is that it utilises both community development principles and individual behaviour change theories. The programme was set up to support the development of approaches to engage vulnerable groups and then support them to make changes to improve their health and wellbeing. The long-term aim of the Health Trainer Programme has been to reduce health inequalities by working with people from deprived and 'hard to reach' groups in order to increase healthy behaviours.

Since 2006, the Health Trainer Programme has evolved and developed across England, creating a national presence to support groups and communities to lead healthier lives. Health trainer services are seen as a key health improvement service working to address health inequalities. It is reported that there are approximately 2,000 health trainers working across England with their local communities (DCRS, 2013). The health trainer role was seen as an entry-level role for individuals wishing to develop a career within public health and the health and social care sector.

What do health trainers do?

The Health Trainer Programme predominantly supports adults who want to make a change towards a healthier lifestyle. The health trainer assists individuals to achieve and maintain their personal desire to change. The Health Trainer Programme works to the principle of informed choice and supporting the individual, while recognising the underpinning influences and factors that may impact on their health behaviours. The key functions of a health trainer are:

- **Community engagement:** health trainers will work with local groups and organisations to engage individuals and groups to the Health Trainer Programme. They will develop innovating community engagement strategies to ensure that those in most need are engaged by health trainers. Typically, health trainers will attend support groups, organise community engagement events and base themselves out of places where groups and communities may congregate.
- **Service mapping:** a key aspect of the health trainer function is to map and build up a directory of existing health and non-health services in order to effectively and appropriately signpost health trainer clients to services and groups. Health trainers will do this by going out and meeting services, finding out what they offer, when they offer it and who they offer it to, and from this build up a map of the local services and assets a community has that they can access. This will range from the local health centres and dentists to walking groups, reading circles, etc.
- **Health information and signposting:** health trainers will often engage with clients who are not ready to change or who are just seeking information on health. Other people *are* ready to change and for them the health trainer will offer behaviour change support.
- **Partnerships and collaborations:** health trainers work and engage with other health and non-health services to provide seamless support to their clients. Health trainers will work with partner organisations to develop effective referral routes to ensure that the client's journey and support from one service to another is a smooth one.

- **Behaviour change support**: for those individuals who want support to change to more healthy behaviour, the health trainer works with them to support them to change. The health trainer provides one-to-one support to the client. The health trainer and client work together to develop achievable goals. The health trainer will then support the client to achieve these. The support can range from listening to the client about their worries and issues; using motivational interviewing skills to keep them motivated; advocating for them in order to overcome some of the barriers; attending groups and activities with them to provide additional support, guidance and motivation.

The principle is to provide a personalised care approach that focuses on empowering the client to make decisions about their health and behaviour, and eventually equipping the client to become, in effect, their own 'internal' health trainer, and potentially even to become a health trainer in their own right.

The key objectives of the Health Trainer Programme are to:

- identify and engage individuals from deprived groups and communities (so addressing inequalities in health);
- enable individuals to change their behaviour to impact positively on their health and wellbeing;
- support individuals to access and make more effective use of health and wellbeing services;
- increase capacity and capability of a workforce with the right skills to tackle health inequalities.

Why are health trainers needed?

> Britain is now the most obese nation in Europe. We have among the worst rates of sexually transmitted infections recorded, a relatively large population of problem drug users and rising levels of harm from alcohol. Smoking alone claims over 80,000 lives every year. Experts estimate that tackling poor mental health could reduce our overall disease burden by nearly a quarter. Health inequalities between rich and poor have been getting progressively worse. We still live in a country where the wealthy can expect to live longer than the poor.
>
> (Department of Health, 2010)

In order to address the issues highlighted in the quote above there is a clear need to focus on public health and preventive interventions to achieve positive health outcomes for local communities. Health trainers are well placed and have been successfully achieving this since 2006. Evaluation of the Health Trainer Programme to date has shown that health trainers are extremely effective in engaging clients from the areas that experience the most inequalities and in assisting them to achieve and maintain their behaviour change goals (DCRS, 2012).

Health trainers and their clients have fed back on the impact the programme has had on health and social outcomes:

> I look in the mirror and I see the same old same old. But when I'm out and about I see this person doing things that make me think who is she and what has she done with Wendy! ... things are a-changing, your work is paying off, is your manager pleased with what you've achieved with me?
>
> (Client)

> When the client realised he was the only one in control of his own body and the one capable to make his own decisions, life is full of choices and sometimes we just need that person to help us realise this. This client was able to regain his life back and most important of all, not to live in fear of having a heart attack and not being able to see his grandchildren grow.
>
> (Health trainer)

> For many years I have lived in a foggy haze, lacking motivation. The support given has revitalised my enthusiasm to enjoy life.
>
> (Client)

In summary, health trainers are key to providing positive health outcomes for the wider population; they are well placed to support local communities and groups around weight management, smoking prevalence, alcohol and substance misuse, and to support people with long-term conditions.

The health trainer role

The health trainer role is underpinned by the NHS health trainer handbook *Improving Health: Changing Behaviour*. The handbook provides an insight into the multifaceted aspects of a health trainer role. The health trainer role is based on four health trainer competencies that were developed in order to build the health trainer workforce. All health trainers will have been trained on these competencies. They are:

- HT1 Make relationships with communities.
- HT2 Communicate with individuals about promoting their health and wellbeing.
- HT3 Enable individuals to change their behaviour in order to improve their health and wellbeing.
- HT4 Manage and organise your own time and activity.

Health trainers can work in a range of settings and as the success of the health trainer intervention increases, more and more settings are being tested out in order to support health outcomes for local populations. Typically, there are three main settings from which health trainers would normally work. These are:

- **Community settings:** health trainers would typically be based in communities, taking the service out to the communities in which they will work. They will usually work from community centres, libraries, schools, and voluntary and community organisations – in fact, anywhere that local people may congregate.
- **Justice system settings:** health trainers in these settings would primarily support offenders and ex-offenders. Probation health trainers would typically be based at probation offices, supporting clients on probation orders. Prisons have also developed some health trainer programmes where prisoners themselves are supported to become health trainers and then to support their peers around health and wellbeing.
- **Primary care and health settings:** health trainers have recently begun to be based at GP practices where they receive direct referrals from GPs and practice staff to support patients around specific health issues such as weight management and physical activity. In some areas, health trainers have also been based in hospital settings to support patients, and in other areas health trainer roles have been developed to deliver NHS health checks.

Within the different settings that health trainers may operate, there are usually four roles that can be seen as a route of progression for people where they can progress from one role to the other. These are:

1 **Health trainer champion:** the primary focus of this role is to work with health trainers by providing clients and communities with information and signposting to NHS and other community services and activities. This role essentially delivers the Health Information and Signposting function described earlier. Health trainer champions are required to complete the Royal Society for Public Health's Level 2 Award 'Understanding Health Improvement', which provides them with a nationally recognised qualification. Health trainer champions may also be supported to access localised training. Health trainer champions are often volunteers and are frequently previous clients of the Health Trainer Programme.

2 **Trainee health trainer:** there is a requirement to complete health trainer training demonstrating the competencies as described earlier. Health trainers are required to produce a portfolio as part of the Level 3 City and Guilds Health Trainer Certificate. As part of their training there is a need to collect evidence to demonstrate that they have achieved each of the competencies. The trainee health trainer role allows them to achieve this. The functions of this role would be to carry out under supervision Community Engagement, Information Giving and Signposting, Service Mapping and Behaviour Change Support. Once qualified, the trainee can progress to become a qualified health trainer. The trainee is usually paid at an equivalent salary to NHS Agenda for Change[1] pay band 2.

3 **Health trainer:** once qualified, the health trainer will be competent to carry out all of the functions described earlier. The qualified health trainer would be able to work autonomously with clients and partners, and should be competent in all four areas of work. The health trainer will usually be paid at an equivalent salary to agenda for change band 3.

4 **Senior health trainer:** not all services have these roles, but where they do exist, they provide a progression opportunity for health trainers. The senior health trainer role can vary from one service to another and there is no formal additional qualification for this role. Typically, a senior health trainer will undertake the same functions as a qualified health trainer with the additional responsibility of providing supervision and mentoring for other health trainers. In some areas, senior health trainers have been employed to coordinate local delivery of the NHS Health Checks Programme. This role is usually paid at an equivalent salary to agenda for change band 4.

What are the key characteristics of health trainers?

Health trainers are a unique behaviour change workforce and have a number of characteristics that make them different from other behaviour change and health improvement roles. These are just a few:

- Health trainers in general are an altruistic workforce; they are passionate about supporting and helping people in any way they can.
- Health trainers are a competency-based workforce. They are trained against a specific set of competencies that were developed specifically for this workforce.
- Health trainers will normally have some personal experience of the issues that face the communities with whom they work, providing them with extra insight to be empathetic to the clients and their issues.
- Health trainers provide a generic behaviour change service, which means that they can use the skills and knowledge to support almost anyone on any kind of behavioural issue.
- Health trainers act as listeners, advocates and champions for the clients they support.
- Health trainers empower, motivate, inspire and guide their clients to their goal.

How to get involved

The Health Trainer Programme is a targeted health improvement service addressing health inequalities, and therefore Health Trainer Programmes only exist in areas of social deprivation. Health trainer services are typically commissioned by the local authority public health team. If the health trainer role is one that is appealing, then in the first instance find out where the nearest health trainer service is and arrange to go and meet with them and spend some time to gain a good insight into the role and what they do. Perhaps consider becoming a health trainer champion for a few months before deciding on whether the health trainer role is right. In looking for health trainer jobs being advertised, in order to recruit local people, local papers and local job sites are usually where these roles would be found, rather than NHS jobs.

Note

1 Agenda for Change represents the standard pay bands used for health service staff levels 1–9.

References

Data Collection Reporting System (DCRS), Health Trainers Half Year Review, April to September, 2013. Available online at: www.rsph.org.uk/filemanager/root/site_assets/about_us/policy_and_projects/HealthTrainers_NationalReport.pdf. Accessed 26 May 2014.

Department of Health, *Choosing Health: Making Healthier Choices Easier*, Cmd 6374, London, The Stationery Office, 16 November 2004.

Department of Health, *Healthy Lives, Healthy People: Our Strategy for Public Health in England*, CM7985, London, The Stationery Office, 30 November 2010.

Marmot, M. *Tackling Health Inequalities: 10 Years On*. University College London, 2009.

2 Health intelligence

Alison Hill

Introduction to this function

Health intelligence practitioners collect, analyse, interpret and communicate information about health. This information can be about the general health and wellbeing of the whole population, or about the health risks and health needs of a particular social group (such as an age group or an ethnic group). Examples of roles in the workplace include cancer intelligence officers, information analysts in public health teams in health or local government settings.

The role is critical in supporting decision-makers across the health and healthcare system to understand the needs of the population, and to identify priorities for action, by converting raw data from many different sources into meaningful information about health and wellbeing to be used by a largely non-specialist audience.

EXAMPLE OF PUBLIC HEALTH PRACTITIONER ROLES FOR THIS FUNCTION

The contribution that follows will illustrate the importance of the health intelligence workforce and the key attributes of those who decide to join it.

Alison Hill, Deputy Chief Knowledge Officer, Public Health England

> In the nineteenth century health was transformed by clear, clean water. In the twenty-first century, health will be transformed by clean clear knowledge.
>
> (Muir Gray)

> An investment in knowledge pays the best interest.
>
> (Benjamin Franklin)

Description of the health intelligence function

Public health intelligence (PHI) is a major part of the role of the new national public health agency for England, Public Health England. This contribution explains why it is a worthwhile career and how to get started.

The scientific basis of public health practice is epidemiology and biostatistics alongside the science of behaviour change, health services management and environmental science. Epidemiology is the study of the distribution and determinants of disease in populations, and is to public health as the stethoscope is to medicine.

The basis of epidemiology is the collection, analysis and translation of data, whether from routine information, surveys or from research, to support public health policy and practice. As it is at the heart of public health practice, the requirements for experts to support both the analysis of data and the identification and interpretation of research evidence have put public health intelligence at the centre of public health practice. This has meant that public health intelligence has increasingly been recognised as a specialism in its own right, and over the last two decades, as the tools and techniques of data analysis have become increasingly sophisticated, and the demands grow for more detailed fine-grained analysis by different population groups, we have seen the emergence of the dedicated public health intelligence specialist and practitioner. These experts, while having an understanding of public health and epidemiology and the essential population-based approaches to public health services, also have a much greater depth of expertise in data collection, data analysis and translation of both evidence and intelligence to create resources that can be used for action by policy-makers, practitioners and the public.

Ways that public health intelligence contributes to improving population health outcomes and reducing inequalities

Evidence and intelligence are the foundations of the public health system. As well as understanding the threats to health through surveillance and needs assessment, we need to know what effective actions to take through assessment of the evidence and cost-effectiveness analysis, and we need to monitor the impact of our interventions. The roles of intelligence and evidence are therefore indispensable.

Below are some examples of where public health practitioners are making a difference through the creation of quality assured products for local authorities and Clinical Commissioning Groups (CCGs, in England only) or other healthcare commissioning bodies.

- **Local Authority Health Profiles: www.healthprofiles.info**
  Health Profiles provide summary health information to support local authority members, officers and community partners to lead for health improvement.
  Health Profiles is a programme to improve availability and accessibility of health and health-related information in England. The profiles give a snapshot overview of health for each local authority in England. Health profiles are produced annually.

Designed to help local government and health services make decisions and plans to improve local people's health and reduce health inequalities, the profiles present a set of important health indicators that show how the area compares to the national and regional average.

- **NICE public health guidance: http://guidance.nice.org.uk/PHG**
  Public health guidance makes recommendations, based on the best research evidence, for populations and individuals on activities, policies and strategies that can help prevent disease or improve health. The guidance may focus on a particular topic (such as smoking), a particular population (such as schoolchildren) or a particular setting (such as the workplace). The recommendations are the result of a rigorous process that is centred on using the best available evidence and includes the views of experts, patients and carers, and industry.

- **CCG Spend and Outcome Factsheets and Tool (SPOT): www.yhpho.org.uk/default.aspx?RID=49488**
  Public Health England produces a tool that helps commissioners to link health outcomes and expenditure: a Spend and Outcome Factsheet for every CCG in England based on programme budgets. The tool and factsheets use this programme budgeting data and overall indicators of health outcome by programme (where available) to present CCGs with an analysis of the impact of their expenditure. This allows easy identification of those areas that require priority attention, where relative potential shifts in investment opportunities will optimise local health gains and increase quality. Commissioners can use the tool and the factsheets to gain an overview of outcome and expenditure across all programmes.

The health intelligence practitioner

The public health intelligence practitioner is now required to have a very complex set of skills. This is set out in the UK *Public Health Skills and Career Framework* (2008), which states:

> This area of practice focuses on the systems and capacity to deliver intelligence for surveillance, early warning functions, risk to populations, measurement of health and wellbeing and outcomes. Practitioners draw together information from various sources in new ways to improve health and wellbeing. The knowledge and competencies reflect and complement the more detailed knowledge and competencies developed by professional groups working in areas of public health intelligence.
>
> The key elements of public health intelligence practice are: collection, generation, synthesis, appraisal, analysis, interpretation and communication of intelligence that assesses, measures and describes the health and wellbeing, risks, needs and health outcomes of defined populations.

As data from routine sources and from research become more complex, and the tools and techniques for analysing are increasingly specialised, many more generalist practitioners now cannot keep abreast of the skills and competencies to undertake analysis or the synthesis of research evidence. This means that the demand for health intelligence practitioners is growing and their specialist input is increasingly recognised and sought after.

Practitioners working with routine data are now required to understand the make-up of very complex datasets such as the Hospital Episode Statistics, GP data, cancer registration data and demographic data (increasingly these datasets are being termed 'big data'). They need to understand the quality of data so that they are able to interpret it with all the appropriate caveats that emerge from big administrative datasets. They have to use sophisticated tools, and utilise a range of statistical and modelling techniques. They also crucially have to interpret the data, to make it understandable by non-technical audiences, including utilising a variety of techniques to visualise and present the data to meetings, and to prepare reports for different audiences.

There is a vast amount of published and unpublished epidemiological research. Practitioners undertaking research or review of the evidence need an understanding of the different types of epidemiological research and the quality of that research. They need to be skilled at searching the published and unpublished literature to identify research that is of sufficient quality to support decision-making. They need to be able to know how to search the vast electronic databases, to filter the best evidence and to critically appraise it. Like other analysts working with data, they need to be able to write reports and present findings to a variety of different audiences.

These specialist practitioners now work in a variety of settings and are a core part of any public health team. People with these skills are few and far between, and it is critical that there is investment in their development for the public health workforce.

Public health intelligence in the new public health system

Public Health England was created (in 2013) to work in partnership with people in the local systems to provide them with the appropriate resources and expertise to achieve their aim of improving health and reducing health inequalities. At the core of this are the knowledge resources. In recognition of the centrality of evidence and intelligence, PHE created the post of Chief Knowledge Officer (CKO), with a directorate that includes staff involved in the management and analysis of data and research evidence. The CKO directorate has eight teams based across England, which incorporated the existing Public Health Observatory (PHO) and Cancer Intelligence functions. These teams are called the knowledge and intelligence teams, and have specialist staff at consultant and practitioner levels working on public health evidence and intelligence. They undertake specialist work on topics such as tobacco, violence, mental health or cancer. They work on the principle of 'do once for all'. Outputs include indicators, profiles, tools and reports.

The knowledge and intelligence teams also provide an enquiry service to the local system, people working in local authorities and in Public Health England centres. They will respond to queries from local partners regarding local and national PHE products, including signposting to available resources and sources of information, and referring enquiries to local and national intelligence experts where appropriate. They support local people to utilise the many intelligence and evidence products developed by Public Health England and get informed feedback to improve those products. The teams will also undertake or help with local analytic work and support continuing professional development of the public health intelligence workforce in local authorities or in the NHS.

The majority of public health intelligence staff in England transferred on 1 April 2013 from primary care trusts to local authority public health teams. There is currently considerable variability in the numbers of health intelligence staff in different local authorities, but networks are developing to ensure that there is sharing of knowledge and skills and mutual support. The PHE Knowledge and Intelligence teams are key to enabling the networks to grow and ensure that there are regular network meetings. As mentioned above, there will be increasing opportunities for career development from entry level right through to specialist, and one of the aims of the new system is to allow movement of staff between the different sectors to ensure opportunities in different settings.

Specific public health practitioner roles in the setting/function and opportunities for careers

In a survey in 2009 (Jenner *et al.*, 2010) it was estimated that there were between 550 and 600 staff working in health intelligence posts in England, then mainly in primary care trusts, or in public health observatories. Others were employed in provider functions in the NHS or in the private sector. There has been no formal census since then, but there has been considerable movement of labour, due to uncertainty during transition and because the skills of this particular workforce are highly sought after in other sectors.

The opportunities for careers in public health intelligence have grown over the last decade and continue to grow. Several regions of England developed entry-level training schemes, which provide for the opportunities to work in different settings in order to attract new recruits to the discipline. These schemes are under review following the publication of the English Department of Health's public health workforce strategy in 2013 (Department of Health, 2013).

The UK *Public Health Skills and Careers Framework* (PHSCF) (2008) has been a catalyst in supporting the continuing professional development of public health intelligence staff. The PHSCF has helped define the skills of PHI staff at different levels and has helped staff identify their development needs. Some staff working at a senior level have gone on to register with the UK Public Health Register either as defined or generalist specialists.

Healthy Lives, Healthy People: A Public Health Workforce Strategy (Department of Health, 2013) identifies the critical importance of the public health intelligence workforce and recommends that PHE and the Local Government Association (LGA), in partnership with other key stakeholders, will lead the development of the knowledge and information workforce at national and local level.

How to get going if you are interested in a health intelligence career

People working in health intelligence and epidemiology come from a vast range of different backgrounds, but the common ground is the understanding of the science of health at a population level, and the skills and knowledge to make sense of data and research, to make it meaningful for those who are going to take action to improve health.

While it is early days for the new public health system, Public Health England has begun planning how to bring in new entrants to health intelligence by creating entry-level jobs for new graduates or people who want to take a change of direction in their careers. The public health observatories set up entry-level training courses to give those interested in a future career in public health intelligence a basic understanding of epidemiology, and now academic courses are increasingly available to provide that early exposure.

Beyond entry level there are many opportunities for career development, within public health teams in local authorities, within Public Health England and in universities. The particular skill set that public health intelligence staff acquire equips them also for other roles within the public, voluntary and private sectors. Beyond entry level, some practitioners have the opportunity to specialise in particular topics, like obesity or cancer, or to specialise in particular datasets or techniques. The more senior staff will broaden their expertise to cover evidence and intelligence, and some may also wish to improve their leadership and management skills. The expectation is that those pursuing careers in public health intelligence will usually broaden their knowledge and skills through undertaking a Master's degree in public health, sometimes as part of a regional training scheme.

Several health intelligence practitioners have now entered formal training schemes, and others have gone through the portfolio route to registration with the UK Public Health Register either as defined or generalist specialists (see Chapter 13). Registration requires a deep understanding of health intelligence and evidence as well as a demonstration of the broader knowledge and competencies in public health.

Personal career

While I had a long interest in public health intelligence and indeed a considerable chunk of my public health training was in a regional health authority epidemiology unit, my realisation of the power of health intelligence to make a difference and to shape public health policy and practice emerged from my experience as a Director of Public Health. In that role I saw the power of evidence and intelligence in influencing and changing the mindsets of clinicians, NHS and local council officers, and elected members was to present evidence in such a compelling way that it made the case for itself. I also saw repeatedly the need to skill up those who acted on the evidence, so that they as users had the awareness, skills and enough scepticism to know the difference between good and bad science. This particular insight was the one that led me to take up the role of Director of the critical appraisal skills programme in Oxford, which in turn led to the opportunity to head up the public health observatory in the South East. These gave me the chance to build a service that combined evidence and intelligence at a scale to support the public health community across the South East and nationally. The public health observatories worked together as a network over the twelve years of their existence and developed particular areas of expertise, and at a time of rapid developments in data and technologies the opportunities for innovation were immense. It was hugely rewarding to be able to lead some of these innovations and to deliver high quality products to users where it was possible to see that the products made a difference to the health of local populations.

References

Department of Health, *Healthy Lives, Healthy People: A Public Health workforce Strategy*, 3 May 2013.

Jenner, D., Hill, A., Greenacre, J. and Enock, K. *Developing the Public Health Intelligence workforce in the UK: Public Health*, Vol. 124, No. 5, pp. 248–252, May 2010.

Skills for Health, *UK Public Health Skills and Career Framework*, 2008. Available at: www.sciencedirect.com/science/article/pii/S0033350610000673. Accessed 13 February 2014.

3 Healthcare public health

Diane Bell; Jan Yates

Introduction to this function

Healthcare public health practitioners are interested in raising the standard of services provided to the public to help improve their health, and in making sure that public health is a safe and effective service. This might include developing specifications and setting priorities for others to provide particular services, as well as commissioning services, and researching and advising on the evidence base for the effectiveness of services.

EXAMPLES OF PUBLIC HEALTH PRACTITIONER ROLES FOR THIS FUNCTION

The following two examples of insight into a senior, strategic commissioning role and an account of a personal journey into healthcare public health. Both accounts show that, when delivered effectively, they can bring significant improvements to healthcare for the population they serve.

Diane Bell, Consultant in Public Health

In a nutshell, healthcare public health is the element of the public health specialty that concentrates on measuring and improving the quality (and, in the context of constrained budgets, the value) of healthcare provided to patients. It is closely related to improvement initiatives, but takes a broader perspective to understand the impact of changes to healthcare services on population health.

Function

The healthcare systems in every country in the developed world struggle to control the costs of healthcare spending on their populations, while at the same time ensure that the healthcare provided is safe, improves the health status of each patient and is delivered with compassion and respect for the patient. Public health professionals have played a central role in supporting healthcare systems in both aspects of that challenge. The public health approach of studying the impacts of healthcare interventions on a whole population contrasts with but complements the focus on individual patients traditionally undertaken by front-line clinicians. Indeed, healthcare public health professionals are frequently said to work in 'population medicine'. In its population-wide role, public health can independently evaluate care, provide constructive challenge to providers and demonstrate to patients and taxpayers alike the outcomes delivered by healthcare both locally and nationally. Healthcare public health professionals tend to be facilitators of system redesign, informing and often leading debates between clinicians on the best use of available resources in order to maximise health outcomes – that is, to use available resources to achieve most for the health of the whole population.

Settings for the role

Public health's influence can be felt and found across the breadth of the whole healthcare sector, including in roles that may not mention public health in their titles or job descriptions. Within provider organisations, such as acute hospitals or community or mental health services, public health consultants have been employed to run clinical governance units, lead medical epidemiology teams and even to run the organisations themselves. More than one hospital chief executive in the NHS has had formal public health training, and in the United States, most successful hospital businesses require their senior clinical leaders to hold Master's degrees in both Business Administration and Public Health.

Contribution

The influence of public health on the purchasing or commissioning of healthcare has been even greater, not surprisingly, with public health teams being based (in England) in commissioning organisations, before their transfer to local authorities in 2013. The competencies that defined World Class Commissioning (Department of Health, 2007) in the mid-2000s in England's NHS included several on the degree of embedding of public health intelligence within commissioning decisions. Again, there are numerous examples of public health professionals who have become chief executives of commissioning organisations, in some cases as joint Chief Executive/Director of Public Health, thereby reinforcing the population health approach to commissioning.

Role

On a day-to-day basis, healthcare public health professionals can undertake a plethora of different tasks or roles, all based around understanding local pathways of care and the evidence base for improving those pathways to maximise value. The starting point is to understand exactly what services comprise the existing local pathway, the extent to which those services are used, the quality of care (in terms of patient experience and health outcomes) that they deliver and how they compare with equivalent services elsewhere.

The healthcare public health professional must consider both technical efficiency and allocative efficiency across the whole pathway. For example, an individual service may be delivering the highest possible quality of clinical care, with excellent patient experience, and as cost-effective as possible – that is, it is *technically* efficient – but if it is not providing care to the right group of patients or there are patients who could benefit more from other services, then the overall pathway is not *allocatively* efficient. By comparing observed patient outcomes with those that might be expected, a healthcare public health professional can determine in what areas to improve the allocative efficiency of a particular service or the whole healthcare system. This is at the heart of understanding the health needs of a population, taking into account the epidemiological evidence, comparative evidence, then corporate and political opinions, first on the elements of a service or pathway, and then on the whole system.

In most pathways in most areas, greater benefit could be achieved by switching resources into prevention and early intervention, and away from high-cost, low-value care. This is rarely popular with those clinicians who are experts in high-cost specialist care, and the role of public health in this scenario is to provide the evidence of relative benefit and return on investment that can, usually, make a clear case for the shift in resources. However, negotiating the change in resource use may take months of dialogue with a wide range of stakeholders, many of whom do not want to see any changes in services, which might inaccurately be reported as 'cuts' unless the healthcare public health specialist is effective in managing communications with the local media.

The breadth of healthcare public health can take in everything from neonatal provision through to frail older people's care. Unless they are in a specialist unit or in university research, the public health professional may find themselves having to be a 'jack of all trades'. The skills required are also broad: being numerically literate, with the ability to understand and use epidemiology, and an appreciation of health economics is also helpful. Given the focus on efficiency and value for money, a healthcare public health professional would also be wise to learn or understand basic business cycles and business case production, and also understand systems thinking such as 'Lean'.[1]

A clinical background in any healthcare profession can be of benefit to a career in healthcare public health; not only does it provide some first-hand experience of clinician–patient encounters, but the shared experience of being a clinician can help accelerate the development of constructive relationships between front-line staff and public health professionals. That said, a clinical background is not essential; what is more important is to be able to articulate the population healthcare viewpoint clearly and convincingly to patients, the public, journalists, healthcare managers and clinicians.

One effective way of doing this has been to translate complex financial data into clear comparative spends by disease (or 'programme') area, such as cancer, respiratory disease or circulatory disease. This programme budgeting information can then be correlated with the outcomes achieved in that disease, such that a health economy can compare its ability to spend low and achieve good outcomes against any other health economy in the country. Such analysis is commonly available in England as the 'SPOT' tool.[2]

Using information such as this, public health teams can identify for commissioners and providers particular disease areas that might be higher priority for early review and redesign – i.e. those disease categories where spend might be high and outcomes poor. Various other tools (e.g. Star,[3] marginal analysis[4]) can then be used to facilitate conversations and discussions between clinicians, patients and managers on the most locally appropriate way of applying an improved evidence-based model of care. Healthcare public health professionals are often involved in such cross-agency work, and they therefore need to have the ability to work with patients and patient groups, and to engage with clinicians of all persuasions, including doctors, nurses and allied health professionals, and with NHS managers, including commissioning staff and operational managers.

Role within the reformed NHS and Public Health Service

Until 2013, the development and maintenance of relationships between healthcare public health teams and NHS managers and clinicians was helped by public health being a routine part of the NHS commissioning infrastructure. The reforms to the NHS in England that were implemented in 2013, however, significantly shook up how healthcare public health was delivered. The move of public health teams out of NHS commissioning organisations and into local authorities or the civil service (Public Health England) may prove beneficial for those aspects of public health that work to influence the wider determinants of health, but for many working in healthcare public health the move to local government felt like a retrograde step.

The delivery of support to Clinical Commissioning Groups through a 'core offer' from the local authority public health team will restore the link between public health and the healthcare system. However, the necessity to have access to NHS datasets and to retain credibility with healthcare clinicians has resulted in evolving arrangements for healthcare public health: some are retaining their local authority employment status but with honorary contracts in the NHS. Others have taken roles within NHS organisations that, from job titles alone, do not appear to be public health roles (e.g. System Redesign Director, Clinical Director) but which, in their implementation, will require all the same skills as described above and therefore they are, in essence, practising population medicine. Some Clinical Commissioning Groups have decided to employ public health professionals directly, in order to ensure they have dedicated resources available to them. This reflects an established model in provider organisations, in which public health consultants focusing on healthcare public health have worked from the inside to improve the quality and value of the care provided. Examples of such providers include several acute hospital trusts or mental health trusts across England. The role of healthcare public health is also relevant in other parts of the new NHS infrastructure, such as in NHS England and commissioning support units. The exact relationship with Public Health England, and its provision of that healthcare public health support, is yet to be established.

Public health in healthcare-related roles outside the NHS

The strategic importance of population medicine is evident from the attractiveness of a public health qualification for roles outside the NHS in management consultancy, the pharmaceutical industry and applied academia. In all cases, the organisation requires skills in considering the optimal effectiveness and efficiency of a system of healthcare for an entire population. Indeed, taken to its logical extreme, it is no surprise for healthcare public health to have a big role in setting national policy, with recent Chief Medical Officers coming from the ranks of public health practitioners. Healthcare think tanks, such as the King's Fund and Nuffield Trust, offer public health training placements, from which other opportunities can develop, including leadership roles in organisations such as these.

Getting started

Those interested in learning more about healthcare public health can do so as they progress through public health training. Most training schemes require placements in or associated with commissioning organisations, in which projects can be undertaken in health needs assessment, evaluation of existing services and the development of improved care. The syllabus for most Master's in Public Health courses will include elements of health policy, which sets the political context for much of the change in healthcare over the last few decades. The opportunities for specific placements in healthcare public health will very much depend on the maturity of the local healthcare system. In theory, placements focusing on healthcare public health should be available within local authority-based public health teams, with Clinical Commissioning Groups, provider organisations (especially acute hospital trusts), NHS England and Public Health England. As commissioning support units become more commercially aware, it is likely that, in many, a role requiring healthcare public health skills will be required. Public health training placements focusing on the policy elements of healthcare public health have been available at some think tanks and in the Department of Health, as well as in comparable government departments in the rest of the UK.

For those already established in a healthcare public health career, opportunities are available to develop knowledge and learning still further by considering perspectives from other countries. High-profile fellowships in this field include the Institute for Healthcare Improvement (IHI)/Health Foundation Fellowship in Quality Improvement, and the Harkness Fellowship in Healthcare Policy and Practice, both of which involve living for a period of time in the United States.

Summary

Healthcare public health can be likened to a management consultancy working specifically for the local health economy, in that it is a discipline that aims to help healthcare organisations improve their performance – and therefore patient outcomes – through the analysis of existing arrangements and development of recommendations and plans for improvement. Healthcare public health goes further, however, by building lasting relationships with the key players in the healthcare system, and working on behalf of the population to make the system operate as effectively as possible. As healthcare systems continuously evolve, so too does the work of a healthcare public health team; the only constant is indeed change.

Jan Yates: a personal account

I wonder how many other people have ended up in public health by accident? I am frequently surprised by people telling me they found the specialty by chance and got sucked in. Perhaps I should stop being surprised now.

I certainly never planned this career; it just found me. I was quite used to challenge, having slogged through a primary degree, teacher training, single parenthood and six years of teaching including two in a school for children with severe, profound and multiple learning difficulties. But what I found was that the challenge was great at the start of each phase, interesting, a little scary, something to get me up in the mornings, but then it faded off. The same challenge day after day stopped being a challenge. I was in awe of my fellow teachers who could still feel that buzz after ten or twenty years in the same classroom. I needed something else. So when I was successfully appointed into the Civil Service graduate management scheme (the Fast Stream) and landed, by accident, in the Department of Health central tobacco policy team, I discovered this thing called public health existed and I was well chuffed.

So why did I like public health and why, after chopping and changing most of my life, am I still here? The challenge I need is definitely there – in spades! And the challenge changes every day. While staying in public health I have had amazing opportunities, met fabulous (and OK, sometimes cranky) people and had to use every cubic millimetre of my brain. In four years or so as a public health manager, working on coronary heart disease, I was involved with sourcing funds for a multimillion pound cardiothoracic centre and eighteen new cardiac 'cath labs'. I worked with directors of public health, heart surgeons, paramedics, specialist nurses. I stood on my desk and whooped when the funds were approved and I slogged up and down many motorways trudging to meetings and consultations in the heat, rain and snow. Days spent with eyes going fuzzy buried in a spreadsheet for hours were interspersed with train trips home with my supervisor saying 'So, if you were the Heart Tzar, how would you have chaired that meeting?' It was never dull, never boring.

Then the Faculty of Public Health opened the door to those of us who hadn't been to medical school; I knew that to really be able to do the job well I needed a better grasp of the theory and principles of public health, to back up the management and education skills I had. Four years of specialist training ensued. More variety. Lots more challenge. Mental health promotion, heart failure, personality disorder, bowel cancer, teaching, eating disorders, board meetings, needs assessment, exams, public consultations, acute hospital clinical strategy, sexual health advice, scabies, data flow mapping, meta-analysis, statistics, auto ethnography. And then you have to find a proper job.

The question then becomes why my current job? Why screening? Why quality assurance? My public health career has now lasted for over fifteen years and I have discovered that the specialty is a very strange mix of generalism and specialism. Everything we do links to everything else. Everything needs specialist knowledge and the ability to widen your thinking to see the topic from multiple perspectives and angles. So the actual content of the job often matters less than the way in which I am able to operate, the people I am able to work with and the difference I can make. I like to be able to sit back and think deep thoughts, reflecting on strategy, vision, direction. Then I like to muck in and get my hands dirty doing something concrete, with immediate impact and direct relevance to real people. I was a Director of Public Health for a while and this certainly gives you a massive dose of strategy and deep thinking, but you lose the time to do the dirty work.

But screening, and QA in particular, gives me all of this. The impact on individuals of one, simple test, is huge. Concrete, real time, terrifying and huge. Imagine being told that your unborn child has Down's syndrome. Imagine your abdominal scan finding a 6cm aortic aneurysm, which needs surgical repair. Then there is the population impact, which is what public health is all about, and to have that impact, the programmes have to work in the way they were designed. We take people who are healthy and tell a bunch of them that they are probably sick. And some of them will get the wrong result. Therefore, ethically, we have a responsibility to do our very best not to mess these programmes up and my QA job is very much about reminding people of this. I get to lead a team of amazing professionals who have passion and skill and do their jobs with humour, common sense and dedication. I constantly feel humbled (and quite scared) that I am their boss and they trust me to take them in the right direction. I have an equally amazing team of peers who keep me sane, balanced, grounded, enthused and supported. My days are varied and often unpredictable. I have a specialism within my generalism and I keep breadth in my skills through teaching and assessing registrars, portfolio applicants and lay audiences.

I work with people I like and respect. The outcomes of my work make things better for professionals and patients. It is challenging both intellectually and practically. I can't ask for more than that.

Notes

1 For more information see: www.improvement.nhs.uk/diagnostics/LeaninDiagnostics/LeanThinking/tabid/93/Default.aspx. Accessed 16 June 2013.
2 Available at: www.yhpho.org.uk/default.aspx?RID=49488. Accessed 16 June 2013.
3 For more details on the Star tool and its uses, see: www.health.org.uk/blog/engaging-local-stakeholders-more-help-on-the-way-with-the-star-tool. Accessed 16 June 2013.
4 For more information on marginal analysis, see: www.rightcare.nhs.uk/downloads/APVR.pdf. Accessed 16 June 2013.

Reference

Department of Health, *World Class Commissioning: Vision, Competencies, Asessessment Framework, Support and Development Framework*, December 2007.

4 Health protection

Peter Sheridan and Lorna Wilcox;
Ian Gray; Surindar Dhesi

Introduction to this function

Health protection practitioners protect the safety of the whole population (such as ensuring the safety of food, or protecting people from infectious diseases and environmental hazards, such as noise, chemicals or radiation) and safety in the workplace (such as fire safety or the safe handling of goods).

EXAMPLES OF PUBLIC HEALTH PRACTITIONER ROLES FOR THIS FUNCTION

Examples of roles in the workforce include environmental health officers, infection control nurses, consultants in communicable disease control, emergency planning officers and screening programme managers.

Peter Sheridan, Consultant in Communicable Disease Control, and Lorna Wilcox, Health Protection Practitioner

Introduction to what we understand by health protection

Health protection is an important part of public health and covers communicable disease control and the control of environmental hazards, including chemicals and radiation threats. Health protection also includes being prepared for emergencies and being able to respond urgently at any time of the day throughout the year.

In Victorian times, epidemics of dysentery, cholera and typhoid were tackled by establishing effective disposal of waste and a clean water supply. These diseases are still seen in parts of the world and are seen in returning travellers. Advice from an environmental health officer or health protection practitioner will ensure that proper hygiene measures are in place and that opportunities for onward transmission are reduced. For example, someone who works preparing food may need to stay off such work until they are fully recovered and no longer carrying the infectious agent.

Good practice in commercial kitchens is overseen by environmental health officers employed by a local authority which has legal powers of enforcement. However, there are still food-borne outbreaks. Salmonella outbreaks can be associated with under-cooked meat, contamination of uncooked or cooked items with raw meat, or using low-quality raw shell eggs in some dishes. In an outbreak the priority is to stop further cases. This may involve stopping suspect foods being sold or consumed. Good kitchen practice and thorough cleaning may be recommended. If the cause of the outbreak is uncertain, an outbreak investigation can seek out which food items were consumed by people who became ill compared with the food consumed by those people who remained well. These investigations may relate to food poisoning at an event like a wedding or conference. Some outbreaks relate to a specific product that is available nationally and national investigations are undertaken to detect the source of the infection.

Some outbreaks relate to environmental exposures to microorganisms. A large outbreak of *E. coli* O157 in a popular children's petting farm some years ago required closure of the farm and changes to some practices. National guidance for petting farms was reviewed and updated, and the arrangements for recognising and managing outbreaks enhanced.

Additionally, the introduction of a national computerised record system has allowed us to detect connected cases from across the country, who may have been to the same tourist attraction on holiday.

Peter Sheridan: my personal career in health protection

I have been a Consultant in Communicable Disease Control (CCDC) for ten years. I studied Medicine at Bristol University and then trained to be a general practitioner. In my ten years of general practice, I was providing preventive medicine through immunisation, screening and managing chronic diseases like high blood pressure, diabetes and asthma.

I became very interested in how we looked after populations as well as individuals. I retrained in public health as a registrar (doctor in training) and studied for a year at London School of Hygiene & Tropical Medicine for a Master of Science degree. I continued studying for the Faculty of Public Health professional examinations for a further four years. My first consultant post was mainly to do with health services public health and I then moved on to work as a Director of Public Health. At that time, the CCDC worked as part of a wider public health team within a health authority and I provided some out of hours and holiday cover to maintain and develop health protection practice. When the local CCDC post became available I decided to apply, and I have worked in North London and for seven years until 2013 in South Midlands and Hertfordshire.

Achievements and challenges

As well as dealing with individual cases and outbreaks, surveillance of infectious disease allows modification of public health interventions in the light of the changing pattern of a disease. Recently, surveillance data showed an increasing incidence of severe whooping cough in young children. This coincided with reduced immunity in young adults and more cases being identified in older adults. It seems that mothers were more at risk of getting whooping cough and giving it to their babies, so expectant mothers are now offered a whooping cough vaccination that protects them from whooping cough and also protects their babies.

Measles, mumps and rubella remain a significant risk at the moment for secondary school children who are not fully immunised. A national campaign to reach older children aims to reduce the number of cases of illness through affording protection with immunisation. As well as protecting the secondary school children this will reduce the overall incidence of measles and protect those children under one year who are too young to have the Mumps, Measles and Rubella (MMR) vaccine.

While we have had some success with reducing meningitis from *Haemophilus influenzae* type b (Hib), pneumococcus and meningitis C with childhood immunisation, meningitis and septicaemia remain frightening diseases and, unfortunately, immunisation uptake is less than universal. Early diagnosis and early antibiotic treatment reduce severity of the disease and its complications. It is important that parents and healthcare staff are able to act quickly and consider this diagnosis early on in the illness. Secondary cases in families occur in under 1 per cent of cases, but we recommend close contacts take antibiotics as prophylaxis – that is, to prevent further transmission of the disease.

As well as changes to disease patterns, we are watching the new research findings to ensure that we are pursuing the best preventive treatments. When an American research study on preventing hepatitis A was published, I wondered whether we should start to use hepatitis A vaccine for the prevention of secondary cases in the household. The old treatment was to give a large volume of human immunoglobulin, which was difficult to obtain and a painful injection. While this seemed a reasonable course of action to me, we needed to examine all the evidence and build a case for a change of UK practice. I led a group of clinicians, microbiologists, epidemiologists and CCDCs who set to work on developing new guidelines for hepatitis that were launched in 2010. Evidence from audit has shown that this has been effectively implemented across the country.

Similarly, new tests become available and I recently led work with another group of specialists that identified a better way of controlling the transmission of amoebic dysentery in UK through using more sensitive tests to ensure effective treatment of cases and detection of asymptomatic cases in household contacts. Unrecognised amoebiasis can lead to severe complications including liver abscesses, so it is important that there is proper follow-up of cases and contacts.

Some old diseases may be making a comeback. For most of the last century tuberculosis was becoming less and less common, but over the last couple of decades the situation seems to have worsened. Identifying close contacts and treating early or dormant disease prevents onward transmission. Sometimes this may require mass screening such as in a school. Detection of cases before they have an appreciable cough will reduce transmission of the disease. Tuberculosis has a latent (dormant) state that is treatable and reduces the risk of reactivation of the disease. Tuberculosis

(TB) is developing resistance to common antibiotics, which is worrying because multidrug-resistant TB requires twenty-four months of treatment. Normally, TB is treated for six months, so patients who will not take their medication present a risk for us all. Legal measures are therefore very occasionally required to protect public health. Public health law covers the removal to hospital of people with infectious TB to prevent them from spreading it to other people. Fortunately, TB is not transmissible after a couple of weeks of treatment, but interruption of treatment can cause the disease to be reactivated. A CCDC may have to give evidence in court that a person with TB is a danger and should be detained in hospital.

Legionella can cause pneumonia. There have been large outbreaks in the past associated with mists of water from air-conditioning systems or from showers. Better management of air conditioning has reduced this risk. We follow up cases carefully to establish the source of the illness. From time to time we detect an increased number of cases associated with travel and these are reported to European Centre for Disease Control. They have a Europe-wide database of cases and can pinpoint hotels or areas where there have been two or more cases, which allows countries to investigate suspect premises. If a case is associated with a hospital, special measures are needed to detect *Legionella* bacteria in the water supply and ensure that the water supply is made safe.

One of our nurses is leading work around prison health and she is addressing a number of communicable disease areas, including blood-borne viruses (related to injecting drug use), tuberculosis, infection control (good hygiene and isolation of people with infectious disease). She recently identified a food-poisoning outbreak in one wing of a prison, which suggested some improper storage of food and consumption of contaminated food. We have worked with the NHS and voluntary sector to improve the detection of hepatitis C and commission appropriate health and social care for them.

Reflections on consultant career

I moved into semi-retirement during 2013. I will miss it. I have enjoyed the detective work of spotting and characterising outbreaks of disease. This requires environmental, microbiological and epidemiological investigations. I try and share this work with colleagues in presentations at national conferences. I am also pleased at having made contributions to developing professional practice and being able to demonstrate improvement through audit. I have thoroughly enjoyed sharing my knowledge and experience with registrars and other members of the team. I feel it is really worthwhile activity whether we lead on local matters or participate in the national efforts.

Specialist training in health protection

Nowadays, public health trainees, known as registrars, normally complete their professional examinations by their third year of training and have a further two years to develop their professional practice to the level of specialist. Those interested in a career in health protection may want to focus on developing further skills in epidemiology and microbiology. They may also want to gain experience working in local teams and at national level. National experts work in a narrow area concentrating on areas such as sexually transmitted diseases, vaccine preventable illnesses and respiratory illness. There are special sections covering chemical hazards and radiation hazards.

For the past ten years, registrars have been recruited from all professional backgrounds. It is required that medical graduates will have completed two years' foundation training. Other graduates will need to have worked for three years in the field of public health, usually, but this not the only option, in a UK public health department. While a minimum requirement of three months' training in health protection is required for all registrars, those intending to follow a career in health protection require a minimum of six months' experience before appointment to a CCDC post. Today, most aspiring CCDCs will have had more experience than this in health protection.

Other health protection training opportunities include field epidemiology training, which is a two-year specialist programme in communicable disease epidemiology open to those with an epidemiology background or to registrars wanting to gain additional experience.

Relatively few current CCDCs are not doctors, but as the current cohort retires (some 40 per cent will retire by 2018) people from different backgrounds will have plenty to offer. One recent registrar, for instance, has a science research background and is keen to follow a health protection career.

It is also possible for UK practitioners with some previous experience in public health to apply to join the European Programme for Intervention Epidemiology Training (EPIET) programme in Europe. Graduates from this programme may apply for UK public health specialist training.

Roles in health protection

Health protection consultants work closely with health protection nurses. Health protection nurses have a range of clinical skills from different backgrounds, including infection control, tuberculosis nurses, occupational health, health visiting, midwifery and sexual health, and some senior nurses have a Master's degree in Infection Control or Public Health.

Some Environmental Health Officers (EHO) have moved from their traditional local authority origins to work in the health protection team where they acquire confidence in dealing with a wide range of diseases. At the same time they are able to provide helpful advice on public health law and the arrangements for managing contaminated land, safe water supplies, air and noise pollution.

The role of environmental health in Public Health England

Environmental health is a partner profession in the fight against infectious disease and has public health at its roots. In the 1840s, Poor Law Commissioner Sir Edwin Chadwick led an enquiry into the cause of poverty. He concluded that people often became poor due to ill health arising from overcrowding, poor sanitation and unwholesome drinking water. He believed improving sanitation was the key to preventing the spread of disease and led a campaign resulting in the Public Health Act 1848. The act provided for the appointment of 'Inspectors of Nuisances' – today's Environmental Health Practitioners. In 1884 he was appointed as first President of the Association of Public Sanitary Inspectors, now the Chartered Institute of Environmental Health (CIEH).

Lorna Wilcox: personal career in environmental health

Modern-day environmental health encompasses several disciplines. I qualified as an EHO in 1992 starting my environmental health career in a pollution team dealing with noise complaints, factory emissions and smoke nuisance. I later found myself drawn to the health protection arm of environmental health and spent many years investigating food complaints, food poisoning outbreaks, accidents in the workplace and ensuring that standards in tattooist and skin-piercing establishments were upheld.

Joining Public Health England (PHE) as a Health Protection Practitioner has allowed me to bring my experience of a Local Authority Environmental Health Officer (EHO) to the role while expanding my knowledge and skills in infection prevention and control in particular.

I joined South Midlands and Hertfordshire PHE Centre in July 2013. The two professions share the same common concern and having the opportunity to work as a Health Protection Practitioner gives me the privilege of developing strengthened collaborative working between two prominent partner organisations.

In Public Health England, we collate lots of information on our computer database from disease notifications and laboratory reports. This requires careful inputting of clinical data by our administration team. The data are collated by our information analyst and reported each week nationally to contribute to national surveillance. From time to time we detect a more than expected number of cases of a disease and will try to identify links between cases and try to find a common source that we can address.

Responding to pandemics or national non-communicable disease emergencies

In 2009 there was a pandemic flu (called swine flu) and emergency measures were put in place to isolate, test and treat travellers returning from North America and some other countries with a feverish illness. Families were treated with antivirals to prevent transmission in the family. Schools were closed and children treated with antivirals for the first six to eight weeks of the pandemic. This may have allowed the first wave of flu to peak at the end of July at a time that schools were closing. The second wave started when schools returned in September and peaked at end of

October (half term week) at the same time as the first pandemic flu vaccine became available. After the containment phase in July, antivirals were made available through antiviral collection points to everyone with symptoms of and for close contacts who were at risk if exposed to flu.

In the early weeks the local team managed all the testing and dispensing, but for the later part the containment was managed in a call centre called the Regional Flu Response Centre. I was seconded to the national Flu Response Centre from October to support the Influenza Surveillance and Information Service. This team developed policy and guidelines for treatment and coordinated the efforts across England, Wales, Scotland, Northern Ireland and the Republic of Ireland. The team also worked with clinicians from royal colleges to ensure that all organisations explained the need for self-isolation of cases, including healthcare workers, the value of antivirals in treating individuals and reducing transmission, and the benefits to people at risk of influenza, as well as their healthcare workers.This was a complex and intensive undertaking. We built on the existing Pandemic Preparedness Plans and have refined the national plans for any future pandemic.

In readiness for such unusual events we prepare plans for major incidents like flooding, extreme weather events, the release of microbiological or chemical weapons, and infectious disease outbreaks. Emergency preparedness specialists devise exercises so we get used to working in 'command-and-control' management in emergency situations, and are clear about our roles and the roles of others in the response leadership team, which differ a lot from our normal style and management arrangements.

New and emerging diseases

As new diseases appear from time to time, we can never be complacent. For example, in the 1980s HIV/AIDS appeared. In 2003 we had SARS (severe acute respiratory syndrome). This was caused by a virus, but once we recognised the major transmission route through healthcare, infection control measures brought the outbreak to an end. At present we are closely watching a new virus that has caused serious illness during 2012 in travellers to the Middle East: it is called MERS-coV, but does not appear to be very transmissible.

Consultant roles

Consultants have responsibilities for training future specialists and other members of the team. As educational supervisors they require knowledge of the curriculum, teaching and assessment. Experienced consultants are needed to act as examiners for professional examinations, as appraisers for colleagues or as independent assessors on consultant appointment panels. These responsibilities are professional obligations and are on top of the day job. Consultants may take on additional leadership roles as formal team leaders as a Director of Public Health, Centre Director or professional leadership roles.

Ian Gray, Environmental Health Officer

Ian's personal career story, 'Making a difference', is dedicated to his late father, Norman Gray, also an eminent Environmental Health Officer, who died in December 2013.

Introduction

When I was attending primary school I used to visit my grandmother on my way home. She was a widow and took in lodgers. The lodgers were always studying an enormous white book and my gran and I used to test them by asking them questions from it. As a young boy this book seemed to me to have the answers to everything I wanted to know about where and how we lived – it told us how our water is cleaned, where the contents of our toilet go, how animals are slaughtered and cut up for our meat, how to keep our food safe and cook it properly, how foul air and even noise and so many other things in our environment can affect our health.

Most importantly, the book explained all of the laws that could be used to deal with the risks to our health that arise. I could easily see that the people who understood these things could really make a difference to other people's lives. This book was *Clay's Handbook of Environmental Health* (Battersby, 2011) and the lodgers were student public health inspectors who, when they had qualified, would be authorised to ensure compliance with these laws that protect our health. At the age of only twelve I had decided that I wanted to be one too. Fifty years later, I was invited to write the introductory chapter for the latest edition of *Clay's* on the 'Philosophy and principles of environmental health', so today's student environmental health practitioners study what I have written for them about our history and my hopes for their future practice! I have even become one of the people who test them on their knowledge and skills as part of their professional assessments. These assessments determine that they are competent to practise. Hopefully, they will go on to become Chartered Environmental Health Practitioners as I am (Chartered Environmental Health Practitioner, number 007) and achieve recognition as a key element of the wider public health workforce. In my view, it is the environmental health component of this workforce that we will be increasingly relying upon to protect and improve our health and wellbeing against both historic and modern threats of infection and contamination, illness and injury.

So, what a long way I have come and I hope you will be interested in reading about my journey.

My beginnings

My journey began immediately after I left school and enrolled at a local technical college where I attended a four-year training course and finally received my Public Health Inspectors Diploma.

I began work in the London Borough of Waltham Forest, but I soon moved to the London Borough of Hackney where the challenges of poverty and deprivation were about as severe as they can get and where, consequently, there were enormous opportunities to make a difference in people's lives. The work could be very demanding, sometimes every day, but was also very rewarding. In those days it was usual for an Environmental Health Officer (we had changed our job title to reflect the increasing recognition of the effects of the environment on people's health) to have a 'district' – a geographical area for which they were personally responsible for all aspects of the local authority powers and duties for the protection of public health. This meant that we got to know the local community and its characters really well – and they knew us, relied upon and hopefully trusted us, at least to deal with them fairly. Until 1974 we worked alongside a Medical Officer of Health in a local authority 'health department', which was part of the National Health Service. The government's recent changes to our health services in England are intended to re-create this original National Health Service concept of a comprehensive health service, of which public health measures delivered through local authorities are a key component.

After 1974, the health services separated from the local authority services, but we continued to work in close collaboration. In particular, health service staff who would be working in the community, including district nurses, health visitors and the new community physicians (to be renamed in 1989 public health consultants), received part of their training with a local authority.

Equal opportunities and environmental health

Hackney was a local authority that promoted itself as being serious about its commitment to equal opportunities and this directly impacted on the way that environmental health services were delivered. At that time the borough had the highest proportion of its population who were members of black and ethnic minority communities (as we described people then) with high levels of unemployment and measures of deprivation. Many people were living in poverty or on low incomes, in bad housing and insecure employment. Now we who work in environmental health can become intimately involved with people's lives – we inspect their buildings, their homes including their kitchens and their bedrooms, we deal with their pests and their rubbish, and even deal with their personal behaviour when it can put other people's health and safety at risk.

Difficulties in accessing housing drove many immigrants to become residential landlords, often buying dilapidated properties and filling them with tenants to meet the costs of purchase loans. Many ran small businesses, often food outlets and restaurants, and they often struggled with understanding and meeting the standards required. Many workplaces operated on the margins and with little regard for safety. The issues of how environmental health requirements impacted on ethnic minorities became a national concern and the Institution of Environmental Health Officers produced a report that identified these concerns.

This was the mid-1980s and I had become actively involved in a range of environmental health campaign groups. One of these was the Socialist Environment Resources Association that campaigned on a range of issues from 'acid rain' to unreported discharges from nuclear power stations. At one meeting we had listened to a man, Tony Whitehead, who had recently established the Terrence Higgins Trust in memory of his partner who had died from AIDS. It was clear to me that this issue had the potential to create a whole new way for ill-informed and bigoted people to exercise their prejudices. Indeed, the behaviour of some public health people, including some environmental health officers, was actually adding to the misunderstandings and raising false fears. There was real reluctance among many public health people to get involved, so I gave a speech at our annual conference stating that we could not pick and choose who we were willing to provide services for. I took responsibility for providing the first professional guidance on HIV and AIDS, which contained a guide to safer sex.

This was the most personally challenging time of my professional life. I became so well known for this work that some people presumed that I must have AIDS or at least be a gay man. It was the first time that I had had my motives questioned for what I thought to be legitimate work, but for some people public health is not neutral ground. I was in good company, however, and I was invited to visit Broderip Ward at the Middlesex Hospital, on the day after it was opened by Princess Diana in 1987, as the first dedicated service for people with AIDS and HIV-related illnesses.

The 1980s – Health For All by the Year 2000

During the 1980s, environmental health had been changing direction with the adoption by the WHO of the *Global Strategy for Health For All by the Year 2000* (WHO, 1981), and the development of a national strategy that made commitments that were directly related to how environmental health could not only protect health, but also improve health. I saw this as a great opportunity and I was soon managing a health promotion team, which was part of the local authority environmental health service but working closely with the public health people in the health authority. Together we were delivering community initiatives such as the *Hackney Healthy Breakfast* and a multi-agency accident prevention strategy.

Smoking was a major concern and in 1992 I made a commitment that Hackney Council would produce and implement a comprehensive local authority policy on smoking and tobacco. This policy prohibited smoking in all council offices and even required that the pension funds would not be invested in tobacco – a measure we are still campaigning for today. The policy was recognised as a model for the public sector and received an award from Action on Smoking and Health (ASH) and the British Heart Foundation.

1990s – health and sustainable development

If the 1980s were about improving health, then the 1990s were concerned with the protection of the environment and the United Nations' commitment to 'sustainable development' through *Agenda 21: Programme of Action for Sustainable Development* (United Nations, 1992). This related directly to our ambitions for environmental health practice and in our report *Agendas for Change* we called for the reintegration of environment and health policies (Chartered Institute for Environmental Health, 1997).

Working at the Health Development Agency

During the 1990s there were significant changes and budget reductions within local government and in 2000 I was made redundant by Hackney Council. Ironically, this was the same year as I had received my twenty-five years long service award and turned fifty years of age. So I had a difficult choice to make – to stay in environmental health or make a 'career move'. I particularly wanted to move away from management responsibilities and do more policy work, which by now I was widely recognised for.

With the encouragement of colleagues I took up a post at the Health Development Agency to lead a project to set out the vision for future development of the environmental health function. The publication in 2002 of *Environmental Health 2012 – A Key Partner in Delivering the Public Health Agenda* has been highly influential in shaping modern training and practice (Chartered Institute of Environmental Health, 2002). In particular, it re-established environmental health as an important element of the public health system and, by definition, environmental health practitioners were properly recognised as public health practitioners. This meant that environmental health knowledge and skills could be properly included in the *National Occupational Standards for Public Health*, and environmental health could be part of the career framework developed for all public health practitioners, the *UK Public Health Skills and Career Framework* (Skills for Health, 2008).

Policy Officer at the Chartered Institute of Environmental Health (CIEH)

My work at the Health Development Agency had been fully supported by the CIEH and I was appointed to a post of Policy Officer to develop policies and practices that would assist environmental health practitioners to fulfil their important roles in modern public health. In this post I have had opportunities to be highly influential in influencing government legislation and national standards in many aspects of our work.

The high point has to be the coming into force of the smoke-free legislation throughout the United Kingdom, which myself and the CIEH had campaigned for during some twenty-five years. It was primarily environmental health practitioners that ensured compliance with the smoke-free laws, just as our predecessors, the public health inspectors, had implemented the requirements of the Clean Air Acts in the 1950s to deal with the appalling pollution from burning smoky coal. The Chief Medical Officer for England stated in 2007 that we had left a footprint on the history of public health. So this would be a good point to end on, but there is always much more to do and my most recent work has been published: the *Tattooing and Body*

Piercing Guidance Toolkit, which is the first national guidance to inform both the people carrying out these procedures as well as those who are responsible for ensuring people's health regardless of how they choose to adorn their bodies – the environmental health officer again (Chartered Institute for Environmental Health, 2013).

Looking back

So looking back, my ambitions to make a difference in people's lives have been achieved in many ways, and I am grateful for the recognition and rewards I have received: in 2006 I was the first member of the CIEH to be awarded Fellowship by Election; in 2007 I received the President's Award from the Royal Society for Public Health for excellence in professional practice; and in the Queen's Birthday Honours, 2009, I was awarded the MBE for my services to public health.

Would I have wanted a different career? Definitely not! Would I recommend environmental health as a career for others? Absolutely – there are enormous opportunities to 'make a difference' now and in the future. Indeed, some of the threats to public health today, which EHPs as part of the wider public health workforce need to provide solutions to, or deal with the consequences of, are as great as anything we have faced in our history. If Edwin Chadwick, the 'father of environmental health', were alive today, he would be exposing the inequalities in health and the unacceptable numbers of preventable deaths. He would be as concerned about the financial costs of these, the unaffordability of the ever increasing demands on our health services, as Derek Wanless reported (Wanless, 2002), as well as the damage to the long-term hopes for the health and wellbeing of our children, our society and future generations, as Sir Michael Marmot has reported (Marmot, 2010).

So, you want to be a public health practitioner? Well go on, work with environmental health and make your difference!

A career as an Environmental Health Practitioner

Qualifying as an Environmental Health Practitioner (EHP) will give you underpinning knowledge and skills in all aspects of environmental health practice, including food safety, health and safety, environmental protection, housing and public health.

EHPs can take their skills into a huge variety of public- and private-sector employers. An increasing number of EHPs work in the private sector in a range of organisations such as consultancies, retail chains and the hospitality industry. Others are employed in the public sector, by local authorities, the armed forces and central government agencies such as the Food Standards Agency or Health Protection Agency.

EHPs continue to build on their knowledge and skills throughout their careers with a commitment to continuing professional development. EHPs who are members of the Chartered Institute of Environmental Health may work towards becoming Chartered Environmental Health Practitioners as a demonstration of their professional excellence.

A career in environmental health ticks all the right boxes for people who want real influence, satisfaction and challenge.

Surindar Dhesi, Environmental Health Practitioner and Researcher

A career in environmental health with research

Environmental health (EH) is primarily about prevention, as the World Health Organization definition explains:

> Environmental health addresses all the physical, chemical, and biological factors external to a person, and all the related factors impacting behaviours. It encompasses the assessment and control of those environmental factors that can potentially affect health. *It is targeted towards preventing disease and creating health-supportive environments.*
>
> (World Health Organization, 2011; my italics)

Consequently, you rarely see environmental health practitioners (EHPs) in dramatic life-saving situations; they will generally be working behind the scenes to prevent ill health and accidents happening in our daily lives, rather than dealing directly with the medical consequences when things go wrong. However, please read on, as this doesn't mean that EH is a dull option. I hope to show that it is quite the opposite.

In England, the local authority EHP role includes dealing with housing standards, food safety, occupational health and safety, air-pollution control, contaminated land, some infectious diseases and control of nuisances such as noise, dust and odour. Additional functions might include imported food control, licensing, health promotion, dealing with anti-social behaviour and enforcing 'smoke-free' legislation. Examples of their work include helping to tackle fuel poverty by ensuring that homes are properly insulated, investigating food-poisoning outbreaks or developing policies to limit the number of 'fast-food' premises near schools and promoting healthier menus. EHPs working for local authorities are one of very few public health professional groups with a regulatory role and statutory powers – for example, being able to serve various legal notices including for improvement, seizure, detention and prohibition, and to take criminal prosecutions. Their wide remit has led to them being called the 'general practitioners of public health' (Cornell, 1996, p. 74).

Health inequalities present a major public health challenge and have done so for generations. There is a gradient between social position and health; the higher someone is on the social gradient, the better their health will be (Marmot, 2010). There is also a North–South divide in England: to illustrate, men in East Dorset live on average 9.2 years longer than men in Blackpool (Office for National Statistics, 2013). To address health inequalities, it is now widely acknowledged that the focus should be on 'the causes of the causes' of ill health, which are the 'conditions in which people are born, grow, live, work, and age' (Marmot, 2010, p. 39). Others have said that 'a large proportion of health inequalities are determined by inequalities in the non-medical determinants of health' (Murty *et al.*, 2009, p. 1404), which means that medicine, while important, has a limited role. The public health professions cannot tackle health inequalities alone (there are many other factors, such as power, poverty, the distribution of wealth and education, which are very important), but EHPs are well positioned to help reduce inequalities, with their work to protect and improve living and working conditions.

In England, new Health and Wellbeing Boards have been established in local authorities, charged with setting the local strategy for health and social care, which includes tackling health inequalities (in addition to other functions) in their areas. My research indicates that health policy-makers involved with Health and Wellbeing Boards who understand the role of EH often appreciate its value in tackling health inequalities. However, many people are not aware of the full range of EH functions (Dhesi, forthcoming).

Where environmental health practitioners work

EHPs work in both the private and the public sector. To recap, in the public sector they are often employed in regulatory positions within local authorities or central government agencies such as the Health and Safety Executive (HSE); but they may also work on policy for organisations including Public Health England, the Department for International Development or the Better Regulation Delivery Office.

In the private sector, they might work for large or small businesses, including retailers, manufacturers and the service industry, and others work as specialist consultants or trainers. Some EHPs have become academics and are involved in research and teaching the new generation of public health professionals.

EHPs can also be found working for environmental health charities in the UK and internationally – for example, Médecins Sans Frontières and Concern Worldwide. The EHP skill set means that they are adaptable and can make an impact in a variety of different situations.

Environmental health skills

EHPs need knowledge of both the law and the scientific principles underpinning their public health functions. They also need to be 'politically savvy', as they are often involved in working with local politicians; and my research indicates that (in England) public health is an increasingly political issue, both at local and national levels, and others have recognised 'the inherently political nature of health policy' (Bernier and Clavier, 2011, p. 114). I have also found that the ability to understand, intelligently apply and contribute to the available evidence base is becoming increasingly important.

EHPs are taught to objectively inspect, audit or investigate; to take accurate and timely notes; and if necessary to gather evidence for formal action, and also to give informal advice for minor issues and good practice. They may need to take measurements, photographs, copies of documents or other materials and in some cases will take statements from witnesses. EHPs have a working knowledge of the legislation and guidance for the area in which they work, and those in local authority roles must work within their legal authority; they cannot simply take any action that seems appropriate at the time.

The role of EHPs, whether in the private or public sector also involves liaison with many other professional groups, such as emergency planners, town planners and building-control officers, fire officers, social workers, occupational therapists, trading standards officers, home improvement agencies, the police and consultants in communicable disease control. Readers will be aware that many public health issues are 'wicked' (Murphy, 2013, p. 248), meaning that they are highly complex and very difficult to resolve, and close links with colleagues in other agencies are needed to ensure that work is coordinated and as effective as possible.

Perhaps the most important assets for an EHP are natural curiosity, an enjoyment of interacting with other people and the ability to communicate effectively with a wide range of individuals from different walks of life. EHPs must be able to get their messages across whether they are speaking to directors of multinational companies, a member of the public who has suffered an accident, a chef with limited English or national and local policymakers. The ability to persuade, build relationships and influence are becoming increasingly important as their enforcement role reduces, and opportunities to take action on the 'causes of the causes' of ill health outside the regulatory role potentially open.

Making a difference

I will describe my own career (which is not untypical) to show the variety of ways in which EHPs can make a difference in public health. I graduated in 1999, and for a short time worked freelance as a contractor and also part-time for a charity, helping to develop health and safety policies and procedures for their shops. My first long-term role was at a rural district council, which covers a large area, in many places wealthy, but also having some pockets of significant deprivation. I worked in private-sector housing and pollution, administering housing grants for essential repairs and adaptations to provide facilities for disabled people, and also worked on a project to bring empty homes back into use.

I then moved to the food and health and safety team where I inspected caterers and food manufacturers, and investigated cases of food poisoning and accidents at work. Being a rural area, I was involved with private water supplies and on-farm cheesemakers, bacon curers, butchers and milk producers, which included dealing with bovine TB, which remains topical some eight years on. At first sight, this job was quite different from my housing role, but my core skills as an EHP enabled me to adapt quite readily.

I relocated to work at a large city council in their specialist health and safety team, which was a very different working environment from my previous role, being urban, having large areas of deprivation and being ethnically diverse. My job mainly involved investigating serious accidents (sadly, including fatalities) and inspecting high-risk premises like large warehouses and leisure centres with swimming pools, and I was also part of the council's late-night noise witnessing service. I was promoted and became team leader, which enabled me to be involved in management, policy and work-planning, and I was able to use the results of my M.Sc. in public health dissertation to ensure that the projects undertaken by the team were linked to the patterns in accident and ill-health reports that we received locally. I also worked on a national project with the Health and Safety Executive (HSE) to try to reduce the incidence and prevalence of dermatitis in caterers.

I was very fortunate in being seconded to the HSE as Partnership Liaison Officer for the Midlands region, which involved acting as the link with local authority EHPs and coordinating several regional projects, including acting to reduce slips, trips and falls in care homes, and improving workplace transport, including the safe loading of large vehicles.

I thoroughly enjoyed this policy role and decided that rather than return to my team leader job at the end of my secondment, I would take the plunge and attempt a Ph.D., something I had always dreamed of doing, but had previously lacked the courage. I was very lucky to be awarded a studentship at the University of Manchester and am just about to submit my thesis on Health and Wellbeing Boards, health inequalities and environmental health. To help fund my Ph.D. and to retain my competence as an EHP, I set up an EH consultancy and have been working freelance around my studies. Most of my current work is in the private sector looking after food safety for organisers of large events and festivals. However, I have also carried out some local authority projects – for example, on noise exposure to people working in bars and nightclubs, and on the control of asbestos in care homes.

In 2010, I was involved in founding the UK Environmental Health Research Network (EHRNet), with four other academics. We are working to promote research and publication in EH, and have run several workshops and written an ebook guide for EHPs on evidence, research and publication (Couch et al., 2012).

I hope I have been able to show, even in my relatively short career so far, that there is an enormous range of possibilities for EHPs and that it is reasonably easy to move between specialism, private- and public-sector organisations, geographically between urban and rural areas, and also to develop your academic expertise. Personally, I have found the opportunity to continually learn new things, meet new people, and to have the privilege of seeing a side of life that is usually hidden, to be very rewarding. To be able to do this while protecting public health is more rewarding still.

How to become an environmental health practitioner

Environmental health is now a graduate profession, accessible via either a B.Sc. or M.Sc. from the Chartered Institute of Environmental Health (CIEH) in England and Wales, or in Scotland, Royal Environmental Health Institute of Scotland (REHIS) accredited universities. In addition to their degree programme, students are required to undertake professional practice, complete a portfolio and pass professional examinations. Once qualified, EHPs must undertake continuing professional development and can apply for chartered status. Further information, including a list of accredited courses, is available from the CIEH at: www.ehcareers.org/ or REHIS at www.rehis.com/environmental-health-officer.

Acknowledgements

Surindar Dhesi acknowledges Dr Anna Coleman and Rob Couch with thanks for their helpful comments on a draft of her contribution.

References

Battersby, S. (ed.), *Clay's Handbook of Environmental Health*, 20th edn, Abingdon, Routledge, 2011.

Bernier, N. F. and Clavier, C. Public Health Policy Research: Making the Case for a Political Science Approach. *Health Promotion International*, 26(1), 109–116, 2011.

Chartered Institute of Environmental Health, *Agendas for Change: Report of the Environmental Health Commission*, July 1997. Available online at: www.cieh.org/policy/default.aspx?id=37936. Accessed 10 November 2013.

Chartered Institute of Environmental Health, *Environmental Health 2012 – A Key Partner in Delivering the Public Health Agenda*, 2002. Available online at: www.cieh.org/uploadedFiles/Core/Policy/Publications_and_information_services/Policy_publications/Publications/environmental_health_2012.pdf. Accessed 10 November 2013.

Chartered Institute of Environmental Health, *Tattooing and Body Piercing Guidance Toolkit*, July 2013. Available online at: www.cieh.org/WorkArea/showcontent.aspx?id=47704. Accessed 10 November 2013.

Cornell, S. J. Do Environmental Health Officers Practise Public Health? *Public Health*, 110(2), 73–75, 1996.

Couch, R., Stewart, J., Barratt, C., Dhesi, S. and Page, A. *Evidence, Research and Publication: A Guide for Environmental Health Professionals*, 2012. Available online at: www.lulu.com. Accessed 10 November 2013.

Dhesi, S. *Exploring how Health and Wellbeing Boards are Tackling Health Inequalities, with a Focus on the Role of Environmental Health*, Ph.D., University of Manchester, forthcoming.

Marmot, M. *Fair Society, Healthy Lives: Strategic Review of Health Inequalities in England post-2010* (The Marmot Review), London, University College London, February 2010. Available online at: www.instituteofhealthequity.org/projects/fair-society-healthy-lives-the-marmot-review. Accessed 9 August 2013.

Murphy, P. Public Health and Health and Wellbeing Boards: Antecedents, theory and development. *Perspectives in Public Health*, 133(5), 248–253, 2013.

Murty, S., Franzini, L., Low, M. D., and Swint, J. M. Policies/Programs for Reducing Health Inequalities by Tackling Nonmedical Determinants of Health in the United Kingdom. *Social Science Quarterly*, 90(5), 1403–1422, 2009.

Office for National Statistics. *Life Expectancy at Birth and at Age 65 for Local Areas in England and Wales, 2009–2011*, 2013. Available online at: www.ons.gov.uk/ons/rel/subnational-health4/life-expectancy-at-birth-and-at-age-65-by-local-areas-in-england-and-wales/2009-11/stb.html. Accessed 9 August 2013.

Skills for Health, *UK Public Health Skills and Career Framework*, April 2008. Available online at: www.skillsforhealth.org.uk/search/public%20health/?ordering=newest&search phrase=all. Accessed 10 November 2013.

United Nations, *Agenda 21: Programme of Action for Sustainable Development*. United Nations Conference on Environment and Development, Rio de Janeiro, Brazil, 3–14 June 1992. Available online at: http://sustainabledevelopment.un.org/content/documents/Agenda21.pdf. Accessed 10 November 2013.

Wanless, D. *Securing Our Future Health: Taking a Long-Term View*, HM Treasury, April 2002.

World Health Organization (WHO), *Global Strategy for Health for All by the Year 2000*, Geneva, 1981. Available online at: http://whqlibdoc.who.int/publications/9241800038.pdf. Accessed 10 November 2013.

World Health Organization, *Environmental Health 2011*. Available online at: www.who.int/topics/environmental_health/en/. Accessed 10 November 2013.

5 Academic public health

Katie Cole; Muireann Kelly;
Jane Wills; Helen Hogan

Introduction to this function

Academic public health practitioners are interested in carrying out research to investigate public health issues or in teaching public health. Many academic public health practitioners are active in both teaching and research. An academic position can involve teaching about public health in a university or college, or setting up research projects to investigate specific public health issues (such as obesity, hospital cleanliness and climate change, but there is no limit to the variety of research) and publishing the results. Research in public health tackles some of the most challenging dilemmas facing the health and wellbeing of modern societies, in the UK and internationally. Examples of roles in the workplace include public health research assistants and lecturers or professors in public health. The generic setting for academic work is often described as 'academia'.

EXAMPLES OF PUBLIC HEALTH PRACTITIONER ROLES FOR THIS FUNCTION: PUBLIC HEALTH RESEARCH

These two contributions come from early career researchers, who share with us their different routes into public health research and realistic aspirations for future careers.

Katie Cole, Specialty Registrar in Public Health

What is public health research?

Public health is about action to improve health and wellbeing through the organised efforts of society. But knowing what to do is not always clear. In some cases, we cannot see what is causing the problem, which makes it difficult to know how to tackle it. In other cases, when the problem is obvious, an effective solution may be harder to find. We therefore turn to research to shed light on the causes of disease and on effective ways to improve health.

Public health research is highly valued by public health practitioners and policy-makers, and is increasingly well funded. It is very broad, taking in a range of scientific disciplines, including epidemiology, sociology, psychology, economics, environmental science and immunology. Some examples of questions that are tackled by public health academics include:

- Does breast cancer screening cause more harm than good? Is it cost-effective?
- When cycling is good for health and low cost, how can we encourage people to cycle more?
- Why does the UK continue to have children living in poverty when it is one of the richest countries in the world?
- What is the best way to finance a healthcare system?
- Can we develop a vaccine for HIV?
- How many deaths and hospital admissions could be prevented by stronger air-pollution policies?
- How can we reduce variations in quality of care for the elderly in UK hospitals?

How has public health research improved health and reduced inequalities?

Public health research has underpinned the greatest public health achievements in history. The discovery of vaccines and their roll-out through vaccine campaigns has led to dramatic falls in death and disease across the world from many infections, including diphtheria, tetanus, polio, measles, mumps, rubella, meningitis, pertussis and *H. influenzae B*.

Academics have also tracked the continuing rise of deaths and disease from cardiovascular disease (including heart attacks and strokes) in both developed and developing countries. In addition to calling attention to this, academics have researched the causes (e.g. high blood pressure, obesity) and the so-called 'causes-of-the-causes' (e.g. lack of exercise, poor diet, smoking), which are in turn influenced by factors such as marketing by tobacco companies and, conversely, by tobacco control policies. Unpicking the complex web of factors that influence health is one of the challenges and joys of academic life as a public health practitioner.

The ultimate aim of academic public health is to produce new knowledge that is then implemented and results in changes that improve health. Sometimes it is possible to demonstrate this success: a team at Bristol University headed by Professor Peter Fleming and Dr Pete Blair were interested in the causes of sudden infant death syndrome (SIDS), also known as cot death, a devastating tragedy for the infant and family. In the 1980s, they conducted surveys and found that sleeping face down, being covered in too many blankets and passive smoking increased the chances of a baby's sudden death (Fleming et al., 1990). These findings were surprising at the time and the researchers needed to conduct more rigorous research to back up their claims. By 1989, their case was strong enough to approach the government's health advisers (University of Bristol, 2012). After a trial to test the advice in practice, the government launched the 'Back to Sleep' campaign, which advised parents to sleep their babies on their backs. After two years, the number of cot deaths in the UK fell by 70 per cent (ONS, 2004) and by 2012, the research has been estimated to have prevented 10,000 deaths in the UK and 100,000 worldwide (Blair *et al.*, 2006; Mitchell and Blair, 2012; Dattani *et al.*, 2000).

While this example shows the power to do good that is inherent to public health research, it also shows that even when the risk factor is something quite simple (whether to place the child on their front or back), it can take many years before research is translated into policy change as we have to be sure that the findings are correct and that the resulting policies themselves are effective.

However, not all risk factors are as simple as the way babies sleep. Alcohol consumption is an increasingly recognised public health challenge and research into its effects and determinants is increasing. While it is clear that alcohol consumption increases the risk of a range of health effects (e.g. cardiovascular disease, cancers and liver diseases) and social effects (e.g. domestic violence, anti-social behaviour, rape, other crimes and work absenteeism), we have been slow to address these problems through effective public health policies. This is in part because alcohol policies are affected by many more factors than just research findings – for example, alcohol consumption is an accepted part of society and generally enjoys public support. Also, the alcohol industry is a major employer and supports the UK economy, so strategies to reduce harmful alcohol consumption are likely to impact on industry profits and may reduce tax revenue. These are just a few points that policy-makers need to consider when determining an alcohol strategy, and that researchers need to understand when themselves lobbying for their research findings.

So, academia operates in the real world. Its research findings will be challenged, its recommendations will be tested and its voice will have to be heard among other, sometimes competing, interests. Nevertheless, research by public health academics has saved millions of lives and improved the health and wellbeing of many more. And it will continue to do so.

Where does public health research take place?

The majority of research is conducted within, or in conjunction with universities; however, there are many other diverse settings that undertake their own research. These other settings often have a wide range of non-research activities too, which provide their staff with an opportunity to combine research with other career interests. Within the UK, these settings include:

- Public Health England;
- NHS hospitals and primary care;
- local authorities;
- government departments, e.g. Department of Health;
- think tanks, e.g. King's Fund;
- royal colleges;
- charities;
- private sector.

What is the career structure in public health academia?

There is no single career path for people who are interested in public health research and many public health practitioners conduct research part-time or enter academia later in their career. However, if you want to specialise in academia, there is a general structure and set of qualifications that most people tend to follow.

1 Master's in Public Health or similar subject

This first step is usually a prerequisite for even the most junior research positions. A Master's degree ensures that you are well versed in a range of public health issues and have training in research skills, including study design, critical appraisal of existing research, statistics, data analysis and communication skills.

2 Pre-doctoral research position

As a Research Assistant or Research Fellow, you will work as part of a research team on a particular topic and may take part in any stage of the research process, depending on your skills. In the UK, specialty trainees in Public Health may undertake research as a specialty training placement or even as a National Institute for Health Research (NIHR) Academic Clinical Fellow, which are designed to support junior doctors to pursue a career in academia. Whatever your role, time should be set aside to help you decide on research interests to explore in a Ph.D., which is usually necessary to achieve before processing further up the career ladder.

3 Doctoral position: obtaining a Ph.D. (Doctor of Philosophy)

A Ph.D. is an essential qualification for a career in research. Typically undertaken over three to four years, it provides an opportunity to create new knowledge or theories in a specialist area, which will itself build on existing knowledge and theories. Ph.D. students spend most of their time working independently, with only a small taught component. In the UK, there are numerous ways to obtain funding to undertake a Ph.D., including: studentships funded as part of an existing research programme; fellowships/scholarships funded directly to the student for their own research programme; and an option whereby staff working already in universities submit research conducted as part of their job for a Ph.D. There are other less common routes to obtaining funding possible too, so it is worth seeking advice and exploring all options. A Ph.D. culminates in a dissertation of 80,000–100,000 words, although some European universities also award Ph.D.s 'by publication' by assessing a thesis comprised predominantly of peer-reviewed publications.

4 Post-doctoral research positions

After being awarded a Ph.D., most academics start their post-doctoral research in a related area. Job titles on the post-doctoral career ladder vary, but the most common are:

- Research Assistant
- Lecturer
- Senior Lecturer
- Reader
- Professor.

What do public health academics actually do?

We frequently hear about new scientific discoveries in the news or the latest policy to encourage us to live more healthily, but what is less obvious is what academics actually do on a day-to-day basis to get to these final products. Often, academics work as part of a team, contributing their own specialist skills to a research project. However, there are key activities that are common to most academics at different stages of their career.

Academic work can be described by grouping activities into three areas: undertaking research, supporting research and supporting others. Activities that fall under these categories are shown in Figure 5.1. At a junior level, daily life will be dominated by undertaking research. More senior academics, who have accrued more research experience, will spend a greater proportion of their time supporting research more generally and in the teaching and supervision of students and other academics.

At all stages in the academic career, it is necessary to spend time applying for funding to undertake research, to cover the costs of the research study and also the salary costs of the researchers (often including one's own). Some academics are employed directly by the university, whereas an increasing number are employed on short fixed-term contracts either as part of a research project or in a professional development scheme known as a fellowship. These are usually funded externally, by research councils (e.g. the Medical Research Council and the Economic and Social Research Council), government bodies (e.g. the National Institute for Health Research and the Department of Health) or charities (e.g. the Wellcome Trust). Researchers need to apply and compete for this research funding for their proposal projects, and therefore an important part of an academic's job is to identify, design and apply for funding for new research projects.

What skills do public health academics need?

While getting good grades in earlier education is a sign that a person may do well in academia, it isn't the be-all-and-end-all. Like most jobs, the skills required are developed on courses and through job experience, so while a natural ability can make things

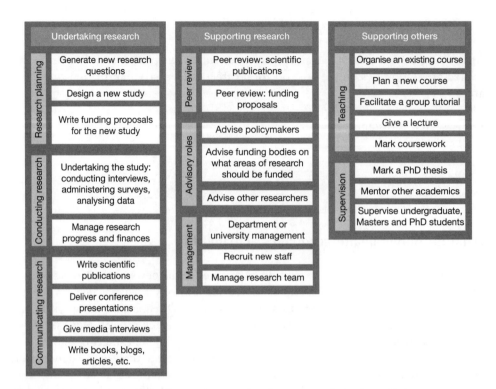

Figure 5.1 The academic job: a schema of key aspects of academic life

easier, working hard and reflecting on your progress is essential to ensuring a smooth career progression.

Academia requires an ability to think broadly and creatively around a particular issue to identify knowledge gaps that could be addressed through refined research questions answerable by a research study. It also requires an ability to plan and undertake research from beginning to end, which can be a long journey with some hiccups en route, so stamina and determination are also key. Academics who read widely and network with other academics outside of their discipline and research interests tend to be more successful at producing high quality, innovative research than those who focus on their research interest alone.

There are many ways to conduct research, so there is no particular one skill set that is required. For quantitative data analysis, strong mathematical skills (e.g. A-level Maths and/or Statistics) are advantageous, although Master's courses will revise important points before teaching specialist skills. Qualitative analysis, such as analysing focus groups and interviews or conducting ethnographic studies, also demands conceptual skills but is orientated towards utilising language skills.

Communicating research findings is an essential component of any academic job, so written and oral communication skills are necessary. This extends beyond presentations and research papers; being able to write for the general public and give interviews are equally important, particularly to reach beyond the academic world.

Finally, management skills, of oneself, others and research, are increasingly important at all stages, particularly at senior career levels. Universities provide staff development training to support staff at all stages in their careers to ensure that staff reach their full potential and deliver the highest quality research.

How to start on an academic career path

In a sense, we have all been on an academic career path since starting school, and continuing in formal education is an essential part of the early academic career. Many of the chapters in this book recommend starting with a formal qualification in public health, typically a Master's in Public Health, and this is the same for academic public health. This offers the advantage of testing out aspects of academia without committing to the career entirely.

Entry requirements for specific Master's programmes are listed on university websites. Generally, universities ask for, as a minimum, a second-class honours degree in a subject allied or relevant to public health or registered qualification (e.g. in Medicine, Veterinary, Dentistry), ideally combined with some work experience.

While a Master's in Public Health is the most common postgraduate qualification, some universities offer Master's degrees in Epidemiology, Medical Statistics, Immunology, Demography and many other subjects that are also valuable in public health academia. If you have a specialist interest that you want to continue to pursue, you might prefer one of these specialist Master's programmes. However, if you are interested in public health, but are unsure of which direction to take, a Master's in Public Health will offer a broad exposure to many areas of public health, with the option to take specialist modules as your interests develop.

Once undertaking a Master's programme, you will be supervised by a public health academic who may even have been matched to your interests. Try to make the most of this opportunity; ask your supervisor for career advice and opportunities to get involved in their research alongside your studies to increase your competitiveness for academic jobs. The summer project, dissertation or thesis offers an ideal opportunity to experience academic life, including formulating a research question, identifying and utilising data sources (e.g. existing datasets, publications for a systematic review or your own data collected as part of the project) and working in an academic environment. It is also an opportunity to communicate the research, ideally through a peer-reviewed publication. Given the potential benefits, it is important to be strategic about the choice of topic and project. For example, if you are interested in undertaking a Ph.D., a systematic review in your area of interest will both help familiarise you with what is already known and also delineate a research gap that will strengthen your case for conducting a Ph.D. Similarly, if you have a choice of supervisor, opt for someone who works in a field that you are interested in and someone who may be able to help you develop a Ph.D. application.

After graduation, early career researchers often look for research assistant or research fellow posts. These can be competitive, so scoring highly during your Master's and having some experience of the research area (e.g. through the summer project/dissertation) is advantageous.

Throughout the early academic career it is important to demonstrate competence, interest and burgeoning experience in academia. The following is a list of desirable selection criteria that frequently appear with early career job opportunities. Note that it is not necessary to have acquired all of these before or in the early stages of an academic career. However, starting to acquire them early will increase your competitiveness when applying for academic posts. These criteria are:

- undergraduate or postgraduate prizes;
- honours or distinctions;
- teaching experience;
- extra-curricular activities relevant to (academic) public health;
- scientific presentations at national/international level;
- scientific publications.

Work–life balance and gender equality

Academia is generally well suited to flexible working with many opportunities for career breaks and part-time working. While much of a senior researcher's day is spent in meetings, at a more junior level, it is relatively easy to agree to a flexible working arrangement, either working outside of the standard nine-to-five day or from home.

The gender balance across all academic disciplines (Science, Arts, Humanities) remains weighted in favour of men: in 2010/11, 61 per cent of all academics in the UK were male, rising to 80 per cent of professors. Within public health academia, however, the pattern is different. For example, at the London School of Hygiene & Tropical Medicine, a leading university dedicated to public health research, in 2010 just 42 per cent of all academic employees were male. However, while there were more women at junior levels up to lecturer positions (70 per cent), only 34 per cent of professors were female. This proportion has remained stable between 2003 and 2009 for senior academics. Male and female staff had similar success rates among those who applied for promotions. An increasing number of universities are applying for and being awarded Athena SWAN awards, which aim to promote gender equality in academia.

Conclusion

Public health academia is a challenging and rewarding career with an opportunity to make a significant improvement to public health. While research can take many years to conduct, and many more to lead to changes in policy and health, day-to-day academic life is busy and varied. Successful academics are those who continually ask questions, challenge accepted knowledge and are aware of science beyond their chosen field. Fortunately, there are many opportunities to incorporate research into any career in public health, through formal qualifications or practice-based research, and this can be done at any stage of the career. However, to make the biggest impact with the highest quality research takes time, practice and dedication, so start your academic career as soon as possible to realise this challenge.

Muireann Kelly, Research Officer

My journey into academic public health: a personal account

Up until about five years ago, I had never really heard of 'public health'. My understanding was that it was what health visitors and community nurses did. It is safe to say that a lot has changed since then. Ever since I was very young, I have been a 'people watcher'. I have always been fascinated by human behaviour and why we do the things we do. When the time came to apply to a university, an undergraduate degree in Psychology seemed an obvious choice for me. The classes I enjoyed the most mainly centred on health psychology and abnormal psychology, and I began to realise that I was really interested in how lifestyle and socioeconomic factors affected people's health and wellbeing. For my dissertation, I looked at the effect of racial discrimination on physical and mental wellbeing within different immigrant communities in my city. This brought me into contact with professors of health psychology within the university department, and I learned more about how psychology could contribute to the promotion of health and disease prevention.

After graduating, I felt that I didn't want to pursue a career in clinical psychology, which seemed to be the path that many of my classmates were taking. Rather than examining individual and interpersonal behaviour, I knew that I wanted to focus on a wider picture. I took some time away from studying and worked in a restaurant while figuring out my next move. I felt that there were no jobs I wanted that I could get with my undergraduate degree alone, so I started researching postgraduate courses that interested me. I stumbled across a programme description for a Master's degree in Public Health and knew almost immediately it was what I was looking for. By this point, I had managed to save some money from work, so I decided to look for internships before returning to study full-time.

I was accepted on the Master's of Public Health programme at the London School of Hygiene & Tropical Medicine. Before returning to study, I travelled to Cape Town, South Africa, to work as an intern for six months. I was worried about returning to study after a two-year break and that I would be starting from a non-medical background, so I wanted to gain some more experience prior to the start of the course. I interned at the Child Health Unit, part of the School of Child and Adolescent Health at the University of Cape Town, South Africa. We were based at the Red Cross Children's Hospital, the largest paediatric hospital in sub-Saharan Africa. My role was varied and I got to do a little of everything, from conducting assessments of service provision in township areas, to writing funding applications, to organising health promotion activities at clinics in the hospital. I was exposed to many of the inequities that are present when we think about health on a global level. It brought to light the harsh realities that threaten some children and teenagers' lives: exposure to physical violence, sexual abuse, environmental contamination and food insecurity, to name just a few. It sparked my interest in health disparities, and the importance of tackling the social determinants of disease became abundantly clear. My time in Cape Town proved to be invaluable experience and was the basis for my Master's project. It focused on government policy around Fetal Alcohol Syndrome in South Africa, which has the highest rates in the world.

My first job in public health was as a research assistant on a project focused on adult obesity in one London borough. The purpose of the project was to explore the barriers and enablers of behaviour change in those with preventable health conditions. This was a fantastic first job and I learned a lot about the inner workings of university life very quickly.

My current role

I am now based at the Institute of Psychiatry, as a researcher on the Environmental Risk Longitudinal Study, which has been following over two thousand sets of twins from birth to age 18 in 2012. The study aims to investigate how a history of stress in the first two decades of life exacerbates individuals' risk of poor mental and physical health in early adult life. This ties together my interests in psychology and public health. As part of my role, I travel all over the country visiting twins in their homes, interviewing them about their life experiences as well as assessing their current physical and mental health, and taking biological samples from participants. I am also a research assistant on a study examining Irish Traveller women's experiences of gender-based violence and substance abuse. Working in research often involves juggling different roles; the variety of my job means that no two days are ever the same. The problem-solving aspect of research is important in public health. Well-rounded data analysis and statistical skills are useful in this role, as well as good communication skills – it is crucial to tailor the message of your research for audiences with different needs and to be able to share your ideas clearly. You need to be able to write for public health professionals, as well as those who are not. Although I am only at the beginning of my research career, my work brings me into contact with a wide variety of people: other academics, public health professionals, local authorities and government departments. It keeps me on my toes, but I really enjoy it. I get a real kick out of seeing our study findings in the media and it keeps me reminded of the importance of research in public health. The majority of people do not realise the role that public health research has in their daily lives, which is the paradox of public health at its best. It is only when it is not there or it fails that we often see the importance of it.

Getting started

I would advise anyone thinking about a career in public health to organise some kind of taster experience, not only to show your interest, but also to see for yourself what it feels like to work in public health. Being proactive and demonstrating an interest is important. Consider all of your relevant experiences, not just formal training and paid work. Public health workers will always be needed. Such a broad field allows you to broaden your own horizons as well. My old classmates are now scattered all over the globe. We are working in wildly different fields – from academic research to conflict resolution, from London to South Sudan. It sounds clichéd, but public health is everyone's business and therefore careers in this field are varied. Job opportunities are not limited to a particular locale or skill set. The choice really depends on your interests. Bearing this in mind, you should take time to explore all the career options of public health. People in public health are very willing to share their experiences.

Keeping your knowledge current is important in a field that changes as rapidly as public health. I learned a lot from attending the free public lectures and seminars that were held almost daily at my university, and I still try to fit a lunchtime or evening talk into my working day if my schedule allows me to. As well as the obvious networking benefits, I think they give you a great chance to learn something about areas of public health or research you have not had much experience with. You never know when something you hear at one of these talks will come in handy or lead you on to another topic you may never have encountered otherwise.

Working in public health means exposure to lots of new ways of thinking and using knowledge, which may be very different from what you are used to. Particularly at an international level, it is important to be adaptable and prepared to listen to the views of others, as well as being mindful of cultural dynamics. Flexibility and an openness to change are key assets for anyone who wants to work in this area. It is important to know about and respect other cultures. There is a shift in mindset needed to change from thinking about things at an individual level to the community level. Having a more global perspective means recognising that there are no 'one size fits all' solutions in public health, and what works in one situation or community may be completely impractical or inappropriate in another.

What I might do next

In the future, I hope to have cultivated an area of expertise in public mental health by combining my education and experiences in research. More specifically, I am interested in researching gender-based approaches to mental health care and substance abuse treatment. I believe that mental health is finally finding its place on the public health agenda and hope to further this development, as well as to improve the health of others through my work. I want to be able to do something that I know is going to make a difference and provide a better quality of life for people. I would like to work at a global level, with the ultimate goal of working in public mental health at an international organisation such as the World Health Organization (WHO).

EXAMPLES OF PUBLIC HEALTH ROLES FOR THIS FUNCTION: PUBLIC HEALTH TEACHING

Public health teachers contribute to a range of specific public health undergraduate and public health postgraduate courses. They will also contribute to students on other relevant degree and diploma courses where an understanding of population health is an advantage – urban planning, nursing, pharmacy, medicine, health trainer, etc. The two contributions are from non-clinical and clinical perspectives, respectively.

Jane Wills, Professor of Public Health

Becoming an academic teacher suits those who are passionate about the subject, either its intellectual puzzles and/or a conviction about its contribution to health. In the post-1992[1] 'modern' universities there are many more opportunities to be a teaching-focused academic that develops the discipline of public health and health promotion, and its teaching methodologies. Presentation skills are essential both for teaching and for presenting. The caricature of a mumbling academic deep in thought is now rare. Lecturers are assessed on the quality of their teaching and on their own students' feedback and dynamism (if not charisma) and clarity are essential. Academic teachers must have experience of teaching and will take a Postgraduate Certificate in Higher Education that covers session planning and setting learning objectives and different methods. They will also be expected to have substantial professional experience that they can draw on in teaching to illustrate how theory can be applied to practice. Typically, they may have worked in health services management, be qualified as a health service professional or perhaps they may have worked internationally.

My journey to academic public health

My own first degree was in history and later postgraduate study was in politics and social policy, so I enjoyed the multidisciplinary elements of public health and health promotion. My route into academic life was through research work, education and then as a practitioner. I had some experience as a Health Promotion Officer and had undertaken a postgraduate qualification, but I also had a teaching qualification and had considerable experience in training and using participatory methods to develop skills and impart information in short workshops. Many academics in teaching universities have a specific interest in the impact of learning on professional practice.

The role

The teaching side of the academic role involves curriculum development, and developing courses and course modules that meet professional competence frameworks such as the UK Public Health Skills and Career Framework, and are at the level expected by the Framework for Higher Education Qualifications. While most courses therefore look fairly similar on paper, there is considerable freedom to teach to one's own interests. Lecturers will prepare lectures and course materials, and most universities now have a Virtual Learning Environment (VLE) that enables students to access additional materials online. Lecturers are encouraged to be innovative in learning and teaching strategies using reflective exercises and group work. Many academics find teaching very enjoyable – it can be stimulating debating issues with students and challenging to communicate complex ideas. Supporting students with assessments and then marking these takes considerable time and marking is probably the least enjoyed part of the role but by contrast, helping practitioners improve their skills and become thoughtful about their practice is very rewarding.

Encouraging those whose careers may be quite clinically defined to have a wider mindset that sees health as a right and to encourage them to redefine their role is a commitment that brought me to being an academic and has sustained me in the role. My experience also made me determined to try to bridge a gap between what I had observed in practice and what I also had found was a dearth of theory and evidence informing practice.

Frustration with the fuzziness of postgraduate education in health promotion prompted me to write my first textbook. Writing textbooks is part of the life of some academics but it is not highly valued. It does not contribute to the Research Assessment Exercise to which academics are expected to contribute and introductory books are, officially, not seen as contributing to knowledge. Perhaps it should be the importance of the contribution rather than its medium that should matter most. It is a highly challenging and rewarding task to cope with a complex audience, to represent a broad area of available knowledge such as that of public health and health promotion, to offer a 'vision' and to incorporate new findings.

Most academics have a role that combines research, teaching and administrative responsibilities. The balance of time spent on each of these roles can vary widely. As a lecturer, most of my work was teaching-related. I coordinated several modules for which I was responsible for the preparation, delivery, setting assessments and marking. With more experience I took on administrative responsibilities, as course director, then team leader. As a professor, much of working life is taken up with meetings, curriculum development and quality assurance, approaches to student recruitment and support, and implementing new ideas. Supervising students is a central part of the role and most senior academics will have several Ph.D. students who they work with. Doctoral studies in public health and health promotion are varied, reflecting the disciplinary diversity of the field. Some of my students are exploring, for example, whether universities can be health promoting, the concept and applicability of critical health literacy, and positive aspects of caring.

Rarely is teaching the main responsibility of an academic and they will also be expected to supervise students undertaking research as part of Master's dissertations or research degrees. They are also expected to undertake research themselves. All research requires funding to support it. Academics may spend considerable time seeking funding for an idea in their own area of interest or doctoral studies, or developing a proposal to bid for an open call. As my visibility as a contributor to health promotion discourse increased, so it became easier to attract research funding and collaborators and partners. Funded projects will normally have research assistants and research fellows involved in data collection and analysis. The majority of such research roles are fixed term and dependent on research grants, and this can create insecurity. Researchers can build academic careers through supervising other students and taking opportunities to take classes, and their hands-on experience can be valuable.

Academics are generally measured on research success, but it can be pushed to the margins of working life, which may extend to evenings, weekends and holiday periods, especially when it comes to writing up the results of studies. Only a few academics in public health and health promotion have predominantly research roles and it is essential to have a Ph.D. Research in public health and health promotion varies enormously in size and scope from large-scale epidemiological studies, such as the COSMOS cohort study exploring the health impact of mobile phones by following 250,000 people over twenty years, at Imperial College, London, to 'Well London', an evaluated programme of local community-led projects promoting positive mental health, access to healthy food and opportunities to get more physically active, led by the University of East London. Many universities work with the public and voluntary sectors in their area in local evaluations that contribute to the evidence base for practice such as that of prison visitors at Leeds Metropolitan University, or of school-based drug and alcohol education at the University of the West of England.

Summary

Most senior posts will expect a Ph.D. and someone who can contribute across all areas. Exceptionally, highly experienced professionals are appointed because of their practice experience. It is, nevertheless, a job that people tend to stay in because it is varied, provides some autonomy and because they believe in what they are doing.

Academic public health is not a regular, nine-to-five job, but rather an all-consuming endeavour that can seem never-ending and can pull you in different directions juggling research, teaching and administration. It is a job that offers you feedback through scrutiny in the classroom and also through peer review of your writing.

Helen Hogan, Clinical Lecturer

Postgraduate opportunities for teaching public health

With so many universities in the UK now offering postgraduate courses in public health and a few offering undergraduate courses, the opportunities for developing a career in teaching public health have substantially increased over the last decade. The majority of posts combine teaching with research as part of a full-time academic career, or with work in other public health settings, such as a local authority.

Role

Most university posts require a commitment to both research and teaching. At the London School of Hygiene & Tropical Medicine virtually all staff teach in their specific research areas and are also personal tutors. Personal tutors identify individual student academic and/or pastoral needs, and ensure that support is provided to enable completion of studies. Tutor roles and responsibilities vary widely from university to university and can include pastoral support only, general academic support not necessarily linked to an area of research expertise, specialist academic input during a specific module or section of a course or supervising a thesis or dissertation. Across institutions, the numbers of students supervised may vary from one or two to more than ten, with experienced staff generally having a higher tutee load. Other teaching responsibilities usually include lecturing or leading seminars on one or more modules related to research expertise. Exam setting and marking may be another element of teaching responsibilities for academic staff. Within many universities expanding distance learning provision has led to the opportunity for teaching to move beyond the classroom and involve the use of a range of new technology such as webinars[2] and podcasts.[3] For staff wishing to develop their teaching skills further, the chance to organise and run a module as part of a degree course provides excellent experience, bringing with it opportunities to develop skills in curriculum development, course planning and evaluation. Further career progression in teaching would involve running an M.Sc. or MPH (Master of Public Health) course, which usually requires at least a half-time job commitment devoted to teaching.

Running a course extends skills beyond curriculum development and evaluation to include student recruitment and orientation, staff development, student and staff support, and monitoring student progress. Building longitudinal relationships with students and staff throughout the academic year enables course directors to identify students with complex academic issues requiring an individualised approach. The Course Director is able to bring together a range of staff who can all contribute to a package of support measures for such students.

Most postgraduate teachers are now expected to have a formal teaching qualification, either at postgraduate certificate or Master's level, and it is often a probationary requirement for lecturers. Many universities run their own modular courses as part of the staff development programme which can be fitted in around other work commitments.

Benefits and drawbacks

It can be very rewarding to launch successive generations of public health professionals into their careers by providing them with the knowledge and skills that will help underpin these careers. Many alumni (former students) stay in touch providing updates on their progress. In due course some return as teachers or research colleagues themselves.

For academics, teaching can have more immediate rewards than research. In a single year, a teacher may be able to redesign a module, change the format of an assessment, introduce new materials to support learning as well as help a number of struggling students gain the confidence and skills required to pass the course. In that same period a researcher may be lucky to have written a research protocol and secured a grant and not even started on the research.

However, it can also be challenging for those teaching public health to stay up to date in their field. This is more straightforward with split teaching–service posts. Many full-time academics ensure they are up to date by providing academic advice to a local public health department, contributing to professional development programmes for the wider public health workforce, inviting colleagues from service public health to give talks and lectures to both students and university staff, or involvement in the work of the Faculty of Public Health or with other professional bodies.

For the future, with the prospect of falling student numbers due to higher tuition fees and pressure on research funding at times of austerity, it is unlikely that universities will be expanding their teaching workforce, so competition for such posts is likely to remain high.

How to get started on a career in postgraduate teaching

A good teacher of public health has the confidence to deliver complex information with clarity and deal with probing questions and challenging remarks, especially as some of their material may challenge students' worldviews or values. The role requires an ability to form positive relationships with students based on mutual respect and good listening skills in order to clarify learning needs and ensure that students access the academic and pastoral support they need. Academic rigour is also vital, particularly developing understanding of advances and innovation in the field of public health as well as maintaining a critical perspective. Most senior educators will also need skills in management to ensure that resources are used efficiently and staff feel supported in the delivery of the course.

The best teachers of public health often come to the field having gained experience in and reflected on the practice of public health in a range of settings. It is also ideal to build up prior teaching experience, including face-to-face teaching, course design, writing educational materials or overseeing implementation of a teaching programme. Opportunities that arise during undergraduate studies might include organising a seminar programme, tutoring junior students or participation in volunteering experiences requiring teaching skills. The professional public health world provides numerous opportunities to design, organise and teach sessions for colleagues or stakeholders connected to ongoing projects. Gathering positive evaluations of teaching from an audience or observations on teaching style made by a supervisor or manager will provide excellent supporting material for any application. In addition, records of attending accredited teaching skills courses are very useful. There are a wide number of short courses available. Consideration of whether to undertake a Master's-level teaching qualification prior to securing a postgraduate teaching post will probably depend on making a commitment to a career in teaching and having enough day-to-day experience to draw upon when undertaking the more experiential aspects of the course.

Notes

1 When former polytechnics formally became universities.
2 An online seminar that allows the teacher to present PowerPoint slides, share other material or answer real-time questions via the Internet with a group of students.
3 A multimedia digital file made available to students for download, which may be the audio portion of a lecture or a lecture plus PowerPoint slides.

References

Blair, P.S., Sidebotham, P., Berry, P.J., Evans, M. and Fleming, P.J. Major epidemiological changes in sudden infant death syndrome: a 20-year population-based study in the UK. *The Lancet*, 367: 314–319, 2006.

Dattani, N. and Cooper, N. Trends in cot death. *Health Statistics Quarterly* (Spring). Office of National Statistics, The Stationery Office, 10–16, 2000.

Fleming, P.J., Gilbert, R., Azaz, Y., Berry, P.J., Rudd, P.R., Stewart, A. and Hall, E. Interaction between bedding and sleeping position in the sudden infant death syndrome: a population based case-control study. *British Medical Journal*, 14 July, 301(6743): 85–89, 1990.

Mitchell, E.A. and Blair, P.S. SIDS prevention: 3000 lives saved but we can do better. *New Zealand Medical Journal*, 125(1359): 50–7, 2012.

Office for National Statistics. *Health Statistics Quarterly* (Winter). The Stationery Office, 70, 2004.

University of Bristol. *Cot deaths: how a Bristol research pioneer has saved more than 100,000 young lives worldwide*, 2012. Available online at: www.bris.ac.uk/research/impact-stories/2012/cotdeath.html. Accessed 27 February 2013.

Recommended reading

For those undertaking or considering undertaking a doctorate:
Phillips, E. and Pugh, D.S. *How to Get a PhD: A Handbook for Students and their Supervisors*, 5th edn. Maidenhead, Open University Press, 2010.

6 | International and global public health

Mala Rao

Introduction to this function

Those public health practitioners working in international or global health commonly work on health programme design and management. In many low-income countries specific, targeted public health projects, funded from within or outside the country concerned, are often more effective than medical services in improving and protecting the health of the population and form a prominent way of supplementing the low level of health services that governments can provide or that families can afford. Health project or programme managers are involved in carrying out needs assessments, planning programmes, fund raising and then managing the delivery of these programmes to ensure that they achieve their expected health outcomes.

EXAMPLE OF PUBLIC HEALTH PRACTITIONER ROLES FOR THIS FUNCTION

This contribution describes the role of a public health specialist working internationally in the statutory sector to bring about action to improve the health of otherwise neglected socially deprived populations.

Mala Rao, Professor of Public Health

Why is global public health important?

The UK was the first country to publish a strategy entitled 'Health is Global – a UK Government Strategy 2008–2013' (HM Government, 2008). Its aim was to encourage all government departments to work together to improve health in the UK and overseas. It also explained that health is a global issue, and that working to improve health worldwide was an essential component of the UK's foreign policy.

The strategy described five areas of action: health security, strong and fairer systems for health, more effective international health organisations, freer and fairer trade, and strengthening the way we develop and use evidence to improve policy and practice. Key components of these areas that are relevant to international public health careers are summarised below:

- Global economic and political stability are dependent on improving health and wellbeing of all populations, as many threats to health security do not respect national borders. The ease with which diseases such as pandemic influenza can spread worldwide highlights why helping other countries reduce their risks would benefit the UK. Similarly, supporting less well-developed countries to address poverty and health inequalities, and the health impacts of conflicts, environmental degradation and climate change needs to be integral to the UK's public health delivery.

- Strong health systems built on good governance are an important means to achieving population health and wellbeing. An absence of such systems may explain why many developing countries are struggling to meet the Millennium Development Goals (MDGs) and rank low in terms of indicators of population health and wellbeing. Adequate funding, which facilitates equity of access to healthcare across the socioeconomic gradient, appropriately trained health workers, access to medicines, technologies and innovations and strategies with a particular focus on not only maternal and child health, but also on non-communicable diseases, in recognition of the increasing global burden of such illnesses, are needed.

- Tackling global health requires strong and effective international health organisations, and the UK has an important role in supporting and promoting the work of organisations such as the World Health Organisation (WHO) as well as non-governmental organisations operating in the international arena.

- The UK is a leader in public health research, and has an important role in supporting research and innovation to address global health priorities. It is acknowledged that at present 'research on global health problems worldwide is underfunded, inadequately coordinated and does little to benefit the poorest 90 per cent of the world's population' (*Lancet*, 2008). Addressing this gap would advance knowledge of 'what works' in terms of tackling global health and social inequalities, and further strengthen the UK's track record and reputation in international research.

An important benefit that comes from working in public health overseas is the opportunity to bring valuable learning back 'home' to the UK to benefit the 'home' population. For example, there is much that the NHS can learn from resource-poor nations about how to 'do more for less', as financial stringency compels the developed world too, to become more efficient in its use of scarce resources. The rising burden of non-communicable diseases such as heart disease, diabetes and cancer present a common challenge to the developed and developing world, and it is shared learning that is most likely to facilitate the rapid development of effective interventions.

The wider determinants of health, such as poverty and illiteracy underpin the burden of ill health everywhere, although contexts and scale may differ from country to country. Women's empowerment and education are recognised as an important means to improving population health and wellbeing in poorer countries, and highly innovative programmes have been established to improve gender equity in access to education and livelihoods. Such programmes may be highly relevant to the UK too, and models adapted to local contexts may add significant value to strategies to improve the health and wellbeing of the UK's most deprived communities, and to reduce health and social inequalities. Public health specialists from the UK engaged in global health have an excellent opportunity to translate such evidence into suitable practice back home.

The settings for global public health work

The wide-ranging areas of action that underpin the UK's Global Health Strategy point to many exciting opportunities for public health practitioners and specialists to contribute to this collective effort.

Global health strategic planning and policy development are the responsibility of the Department of Health, and opportunities may be available for public health specialists to become involved as advisers to support this function. However, the Department for International Development (DFID) takes the lead responsibility for many global health areas of action, ranging from food security strategies to strengthening health systems to achieve the MDGs (HM Government, 2011). Other Government Departments also have health responsibilities such as the Ministry of Defence in reducing the health impacts of conflict, and the Department for Energy and Climate Change in supporting the poorest countries to mitigate the health impacts of climate change. There is potential for public health specialists with appropriate training to be involved in all these areas of work, but DFID has been a particularly sought-after destination for public health specialists committed to working in the global health sector.

The World Health Organization (WHO) is the specialised agency of the United Nations concerned with international public health, but other parts of the UN, such as the Food and Agricultural Organization, United Nation's Children's Fund and the World Bank, are also involved in public health. Non-governmental organisations engaged in a variety of public health activities, such as Médecins Sans Frontières, an international medical and humanitarian aid organisation, and Oxfam International, which fights against poverty and injustice, also offer interesting and fulfilling opportunities for public health work. Working for these international agencies usually requires working in other countries in settings that may include government departments, hospitals, primary care units and refugee camps.

Within the UK, NHS institutions such as the National Institute for Health and Care Excellence (NICE) as well as the Health Protection agency may have global responsibilities, such as, in the case of NICE, to support health technology assessments, and in the case of health protection organisations, disease surveillance and emergency preparedness. Centres for disease surveillance and control – for example, in Europe – also offer opportunities for public health specialists with appropriate training.

Academic public health departments have a significant role to play in enhancing the research capacity of developing countries and in encouraging evidence-based public health practice through research collaborations. They also have a role in capacity building through partnerships in training and education. Increasingly, the trend is for UK universities to establish overseas campuses, where many more learners from the host country can participate in academic programmes, and more UK researchers and teachers have an opportunity to contribute to global work.

It is also not uncommon for public health specialists and practitioners to join one of the well-established consultancy organisations that are often engaged in large and complex projects, such as transforming a country's or state's entire health delivery system.

The aptitudes, skills and qualifications required to be a successful global public health worker

Working in international public health can be a richly rewarding experience for individuals with the appropriate skills, attitudes and interest. However, working in new, culturally very unfamiliar and often resource-constrained environments can be challenging.

Public health specialist training is a crucial first step towards acquiring the competences and skills that would enable an individual to make a difference. The UK public health specialist core competencies are in:

- the surveillance and assessment of the population's health and wellbeing;
- assessing the evidence of effectiveness of interventions, programmes and services to improve population health and wellbeing;
- policy and strategy development and implementation for population health and wellbeing; and
- leadership and collaborative working for population health and wellbeing

These are as essential to be an effective contributor to global public health as to public health in the UK. The five *defined* competency areas of health improvement, health protection, public health intelligence, academic public health, and health and social care quality add value if an individual is particularly interested in a career in global public health research or communicable disease control, for example.

However, the right attitudes are probably even more important. Working overseas is often not easy. Cultural sensitivity and the flexibility and resilience to adapt to physical discomforts such as having to work in harsh climates, and in areas with poor access to potable water, sanitation and electricity, for example, are determinants of a successful career in global public health. A positive mindset, a spirit of enquiry and understanding that we have much to learn from the poorest communities, and a deep commitment to working with the world's poor are key to an enjoyable and satisfying career in global public health.

Examples of where public health people have made a difference

Britain has a proud history of involvement in global public health. Sir Ronald Ross was a British doctor who won the Nobel Prize in Medicine for his discovery of the malarial parasite and how malaria was transmitted, through extensive public health research carried out in India and other parts of the world. Many of the best systems for health surveillance and research in the developing world were established by pioneers in global health from the UK.

A more contemporary example is that of non-governmental organisations founded in the UK, such as Oxfam, which have established themselves as among the most respected, knowledgeable and politically influential organisations engaged in public health action around the world.

My journey

Following a twenty-seven-year career in public health in England, I myself had the opportunity, under the aegis of the UK 'Health is Global' strategy, to establish the Public Health Foundation of India's first Institute of Public Health as its founding Director from 2008 to 2011.

Although UK universities have an abundance of research collaborations that have strengthened India's public health research capacity, there remains a significant gap in terms of competence and skills necessary for public health practice and delivery. I was delighted to have the opportunity to put to good use my own UK public health specialist training and experience, and among the first training programmes that I established were those intended to strengthen the core skills of District Medical Officers whose roles are not dissimilar to those of UK Directors of Public Health. I also discovered striking similarities in terms of the complex problems the UK and Indian systems were trying to grapple with, such as how best to provide evidence-based healthcare to their populations against a background of finite budgets. Such shared challenges gave me an ideal opportunity to catalyse, to mutual benefit, collaborations between the best of the NHS institutions such as NICE, which has been transformational in driving greater effectiveness and efficiency in the NHS, and their Indian counterparts.

In India, millions cannot access health services because they cannot afford the direct payments required at the point of delivery, and where people do access services they often incur catastrophic costs, which destroy their livelihoods. The nation's aspiration to introduce universal health coverage and establish equity of access to healthcare was another major area of transformation to which I could contribute my public health skills and experience in healthcare priority setting and commissioning.

Among the most satisfying achievements of my career is the support I have been able to provide to Madhya Pradesh, one of the poorest states of India, in strengthening its health financing models and pathways to deliver care. Millions of the poorest people in the state are likely to have benefited as a result of these reforms, and it is humbling to know that opportunities to deliver such transformational changes are available to those of us who wish to take them.

How to get going if you are interested in the field of international public health

The first thing to do is to get to know something about the major organisations engaged in public health. Surfing the Internet is a good way to start, as their websites often provide excellent information on their core areas of work and opportunities for employment. Customised e-resources designed to meet the needs of public health practitioners and specialists in the UK, such as the UK Public Health Careers website (www.phorcast.org.uk), also offers useful information on global organisations worth exploring.[1] Joining an organisation such as MEDSIN, a students' network engaged in global health is an ideal way to meet like-minded individuals and be updated on opportunities for work. Internships and short assignments are also helpful as 'tasters' and in determining the best fit for individuals aspiring to long-term careers in global public health.

Note

1   www.phorcast.org.uk/page.php?area_id=2. Accessed 29 April 2013.

References

European Programme for Intervention Epidemiology Training (EPIET). Available online at: http://ecdc.europa.eu/en/epiet/Pages/HomeEpiet.aspx. Accessed 10 November 2013.

HM Government. *Health is Global: A UK Government Strategy 2008–2013*. London, 30 September 2008. Available online at: www.dh.gov.uk/en/Publicationsandstatistics/Publi cations/PublicationsPolicyAndGuidance/DH_088702. Accessed 10 November 2013.

HM Government. *Health is Global: An Outcomes Framework for Global Health 2011–2015*. London, March 2011. Available online at: www.gov.uk/government/uploads/ system/uploads/attachment_data/file/67578/health-is-global.pdf. Accessed 10 November 2013.

Primorolo D, Malloch-Brown, M. and Lewis, I. Health is global: a UK Government strategy for 2008–2013.*The Lancet*, 373, 9662, 443–445. 2009.

Part 3

Settings for public health practice
Fiona Sim and Jenny Wright

This part presents a series of personal accounts from public health practitioners about what it is like to undertake public health work from different settings.

The settings for delivering public health in this part are:

- local authority
- health services
- policy
- international and global health
- voluntary and community (third) sector.

7 | Local authorities

Anita Parkin; Clare Ebberson,
Martin Seymour and Rebecca Hams

Introduction to this setting

Local councils are led by elected councillors who are voted for by local people. Advised by paid officials, councillors make the major decisions on the services the council provides, oversee how those services are run and represent the interests of people in their division or ward (the area they are elected to represent). They are normally elected every four years in local elections. This element of democracy is key, ensuring public accountability and scrutiny, and distinguishes councils from some other public bodies, such as the NHS.

Local authorities have a wide range of powers and duties. These vary between type of local authority – for example, a county council's duties are different from a district or town council. Unitary authorities (as their name implies) carry out all the required functions. National policy is set by central government, but local councils are responsible for all day-to-day services and local matters. They are mainly funded by the government's revenue support grant, council tax and redistributed business rates. The responsibilities of councils are very wide and include:

- education
- environment including parks and green spaces
- housing
- leisure and culture (including County Sports Partnerships)
- environmental health
- trading Standards
- roads and transport
- planning
- social care
- community safety
- economic development.

Since 1 April 2013, in England as a result of the Health and Social Care Act 2012, upper tier councils (that is, county councils and unitary authorities) have new public health commissioning and strategic responsibilities, and employ public health teams to deliver them.

When reading this chapter it should be noted that, although public health has always been important to local government, these roles are quite new, only established formally since April 2013. While the descriptions of the recent changes may indicate some uncertainties, it is also an exciting time to enter and become part of the new and evolving public health service.

EXAMPLES OF PUBLIC HEALTH ROLES IN THIS SETTING

The two contributors cover what it is like to deliver public health roles within local government and describe the enormous potential to improve population health from this setting.

Anita Parkin, Director of Public Health

Introduction

The Health and Social Care Act 2012 mandated the establishment of Health and Wellbeing Boards as statutory committees of local authorities charged with ensuring improvement in the health of the local population; one direct consequence of the act was to move a substantial part of the NHS public health function to local authorities in England, effective since April 2013. The network of public health services provided by the NHS, local authorities, and the private and voluntary sector all commissioned by local authority public health teams require these teams to have a strong pool of public health skills and knowledge.

Although fundamentally a massive change, some things don't change. Regardless of setting, fundamentally the public health role remains overall to improve health, prevent disease and reduce health inequalities; ensure high quality, equitable and evidence-based health and social care; protect the health of the public; maximise the potential and contribution of the public health community; promote better health and better healthcare. However, the context is very different in local government. Public health has a strong strategic role in matters relating to health, public health, and a key role as a member of the Health and Wellbeing Board.

The environment is very different from before (in the NHS), focusing on the elected members as the representatives of the community and indeed representing the community on a variety of issues, wider than health but all fundamentally relating to the wider determinants of health. There is a clear message that public health must continue to work with the new NHS Clinical Commissioning Groups (CCGs) and the Director of Public Health has a clear role facilitating relationships between local government and both providers (NHS Trusts) and Commissioners (CCGs) in the NHS.

Health and Wellbeing Boards have a key role in developing effective ways of joint working. This opportunity needs to be grasped, as it is pivotal and potentially powerful. They need to clearly define the population and agree outcomes; this should be embodied in the joint health and wellbeing strategy. Clearly, the Director of Public Health has been given rights to be part of the leadership of this. With these rights come responsibilities for all public health and all partners, and the buck stops here: the Health and Wellbeing Board.

There are opportunities and freedoms, but clearly implications resulting from the changes and the new system. There are more opportunities for influencing the selection of interventions and outcomes for public health, and the putting in place of systems-wide approaches. The changed system is complex and part of the new skills required are to understand and relish working with this complexity.

One of the main challenges of the recently reformed system that will hopefully be resolved with time is that the public health workforce is poorly defined and very complex, as it includes individuals from diverse backgrounds such as epidemiologists and community nurses. Dedicated public health resources are scarce and dispersed across a range of organisations. The front-line delivery system for public health includes staff within local government, the third sector, wider community health and 'any willing provider' to the NHS.

Public health practitioner role

Public health practitioners are key members of the public health workforce and can have a great influence on the health and wellbeing of individuals, groups, communities and populations. They work across the full breadth of public health from health improvement and health protection, to health information, community development and nutrition, in a wide range of settings in local government.

The role of a public health practitioner can contribute to a range of strategies – for example, planning, developing and implementing delivery of a partnership programme; initiatives to improve health and wellbeing over several different sectors and settings; understanding and being able to communicate the key elements of national strategies; being able to offer specialist advice within areas of expertise and experience. The context can therefore be very diverse and flexibility is a key attribute.

Three broad themes differentiate the public health practitioner from the generic healthcare workforce. These are the clear focus on health rather than illness, the role of change agent and the role to facilitate outcome-focused delivery. Practitioners are generally concerned with a social model of health rather than a disease model, including looking at life circumstances, public participation, health improvement and community development. There is a clear link between a strategic approach to public health and a more operational approach, building partnerships and achieving outcomes.

The main purpose of the public health practitioner is to provide a visible focus for the development, commissioning and delivery of opportunistic and planned interventions for improving or protecting the health and wellbeing of the local population.

This includes working with other practitioners from a wide variety of disciplines, including education, social care, housing, benefits, as well as the more familiar settings such as primary and secondary care. Core areas of work include supporting the development and inclusion of public health interventions by working with others inside and outside the local authority, and with NHS partners and the local community.

Specific public health practitioner skills needed in local government settings

A typical day for a public health practitioner will involve: telephone calls, making site visits, partnership working, presentations, meetings (external partnerships and internal team), and reviewing and advising on health improvement initiatives or actions. The most important skills and knowledge required for this type of work are communication skills, public health knowledge, project management skills and partnership development skills. Some of the characteristics that make a successful public health practitioner include being open-minded. Public health is so broad and interacts in so many different ways with different people and groups that you need to be flexible in order to engage with people. Being committed to the role at times is not easy and it can be frustrating. It is important to keep delivering and supporting the population groups when at times other pressures could draw you away. A public health practitioner will be a 'people person'. As they work with people in many different roles, it is crucial to enjoy meeting and working with people to be effective. In public health you need to keep focused on the big picture, without losing the local context.

Getting started

There are a variety of routes into practitioner roles and probably no two are the same in a local authority setting. You can enter following many types of experience and qualifications, including any combination of management experience or qualification, project management experience, basic or more advanced qualification in public health practice, and so on. Life experience and the self-awareness and insight to see their transferable relevance combined with a genuine interest and desire to be involved with a public health role are important factors in deciding that a public health career is the direction to choose.

If I were advising someone considering working in a public health practitioner role, I would suggest that they should first get the basic qualifications to understand the theory of public health and the many options that are contained within a career in public health. I would also suggest that they back this up with a range of experiences or jobs that help support the knowledge and, where there is the opportunity, to apply it in real settings. (These experiences or roles may not directly link in to traditional public health roles.) Using this route there needs to be a clear motivation to work to make a difference, even if the results from the population data may not be discernible in the short term.

Challenges, benefits and rewards of working in this setting

Part of the public health role in local authorities is to support them to make the best decisions, and the Director of Public Health has a key strategic role in this. This will need a new business model for public health, requiring a change in language and approach. There is a greater need for skills in translating complex information and evidence into meaningful recommendations than ever before. The local NHS commissioners also need pragmatic solutions based on the best evidence available, and support from public health about the implications and impact of different commissioning decisions. Public health will continue to be an advocate for health and provides an advisory service to NHS commissioning functions rather than being an empire in its own right. There is a change in style, one that is more facilitative and seeks outcome delivery through others. This transformation will not have taken place overnight with the move to local government. There will need to be help and support in adapting people to function in the new system and different opportunities at different stages in the workforce development process.

Public health outcomes delivery does not rest with a relatively small public health workforce. More people will recognise that they have core public health skills and the public health team has a key part to play in facilitating a new style of working and empowering others to take on leadership roles for health. The traditional NHS model of public health as the sole advocate and the Director of Public Health as the champion for health must be consigned to the past, with a new conceptual model for the new environment with public health working corporately in the local authority.

Local authorities have a wide variety of staff working in front-line roles and facilitating front-line delivery of public health interventions among their other roles. These include traditional health improvement roles, such as tobacco control, obesity, sexual health, and drugs and alcohol roles, but also a wide range of the more generic health and wellbeing roles. The real challenge here is to ensure that practitioners are able to assert their public health role among other tasks and ensure that the whole public health offer across the council, if not integrated, is coherent and understood by the workforce, politicians, the third sector and the NHS. Perhaps one of the biggest hurdles when defining the role of a public health practitioner is the perception of the practitioner him- or herself.

For example, in a council, does a youth worker who works primarily with young people educating them about sexual health issues see themselves as a public health practitioner, or a youth worker, or both? It sounds clichéd to say that you want a job that could make a difference to people and improve things, but it must be in a way that is supportive and not dictatorial. However, this is a useful concept to examine as it needs to extend to being able to enable and facilitate other workers and community members to capitalise on their opportunities to 'make every contact count', not only undertaking their own defined or statutory role but being aware and able to communicate public health messages.

The role of public health practitioners is changing with the move to local government – for example, a tobacco control team extending its role to work with Trading Standards in the area of illicit tobacco control; work on the health issues of shisha pipe use in shisha lounges, and the risks of shisha tobacco smoking; and working more closely with the media and elected members (councillors) to raise awareness. Public health practitioners work in areas such as the reduction of infant mortality (preventing deaths in babies under one year old), conventionally by supporting breast feeding and the prevention of smoking in pregnancy, but also working with community and religious communities, for example, to support the development of raised awareness and community-based information relating to the genetic risks of first-cousin marriages. Practitioners are supporting work in accessing welfare benefits advice, working with the third sector, children's centres, primary care, to extend provision in settings where people are already receiving services or where they are likely to visit. This type of change clearly shows that in the environment of the local authority there is a growing opportunity to influence the wider determinants of health.

My own career path

My original background is in academic statistics and health economics. I worked subsequently in the NHS in various information, performance and public health intelligence roles in various incarnations of the NHS in area and district health authorities, public health observatories, primary care groups and primary care trusts[1] in various parts of England. When it became possible from 2003 as a non-medic to qualify in public health as a specialist, I successfully submitted a retrospective portfolio of my work and qualifications to the UK Public Health Register. I have since worked as a Director of Public Health, appointed jointly between NHS and local government, with two different local authorities, first in the South East and then in the North of England.

Clare Ebberson, Martin Seymour and Rebecca Hams, Specialty Registrars in Public Health

Local authorities in England are the setting in which local public health teams have been based since April 2013. Local authorities have responsibility for a defined geographic area, with public health teams being responsible for the public health needs of individuals in that area. Between 1974 and April 2013, local public health teams in England had been based in the NHS, latterly in NHS Primary Care Trusts. Following the period of upheaval to new local, regional and national structures, public health is now settling into its new settings and structures, with local authorities being home for local public health teams.

Local authorities have a wide range of roles and responsibilities in a local area, many of which can impact on the health and wellbeing of the local population, either positively or negatively, and either directly or indirectly. Indeed, local government has its foundations in public health, in health protection and health improvement, from its early beginnings in the nineteenth century, and while many of the health challenges of the twenty-first century might be very different, the contribution of local government today to improve health and address inequities in health is equally important. Most of the areas in which local authorities have a role have been listed above.

Campbell's (2010) adaptation of Dahlgren and Whitehead's health map is below and outlines some of the ways in which local government can make a difference in influencing areas that contribute to individuals' and community health and wellbeing.

Local authorities have been described as 'a shaper of place'. Their influence goes much wider than the direct services they provide – for example, through their regulatory

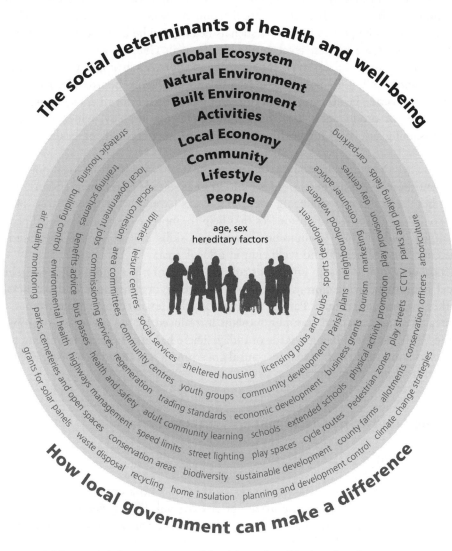

Figure 7.1 The social determinants of health and wellbeing: local government contribution

Source: Reproduced with kind permission of the Local Government Association (www.local.gov.uk)

and licensing roles they can influence the availability of fast foods or alcohol, and hence impact on what we all eat or drink. The wider consequences of local authority actions also impact for better or worse on public health and inequalities – for example, designing local areas (or improving existing areas) so that there are safe, clean and well-lit parks, walkways and cycle paths can influence the amount of healthy physical activity that people take. Likewise, implementing 20mph speed restrictions in residential areas has been shown to reduce injuries due to road traffic accidents, particularly those involving pedestrians, and increase the 'walkability' of an area.

Decisions in local authorities are made by councillors who are elected by the local community to represent their area. Specific councillors may be given responsibility (a portfolio) for leading on certain areas such as health, and he or she will then represent public health at the highest level within the council. Council services are managed and run by council officers who report to councillors. Each upper tier and unitary local authority is required to have a Health and Wellbeing Board. The role of this board is to oversee healthcare, social care and public health locally. The board is also responsible for producing a local health and wellbeing strategy, which sets out the commissioning priorities for health and social care services and for health improvement.

Public health teams contribute to assessing the health needs of the local population and contribute to the production of a Joint Strategic Needs Assessment (JSNA), which describes the health and wellbeing needs *and* assets (strengths) in a local area. Health and wellbeing assets are any resources that help to improve the health of local people. Examples could include community knowledge, skills and voluntary organisations that contribute to health and wellbeing in a local area.

Local government has an important role as leaders of place and local partnerships. Local authorities work closely with a wide range of organisations and partnership working is very important. Partnership working has evolved over time from Local Strategic Partnerships and community plans introduced by the previous government, to the Health and Wellbeing Boards of today. There has also been an increasing focus on localism in recent years, whereby central government has aimed to transfer decisions to local level and communities.

'One-tier' or 'two-tier' local authority arrangements

Two-tier areas

In a local area with 'two-tier' arrangements, there is both a county council and also one of the following: a district, borough or city council. In two-tier areas, the county council delivers services such as planning, education, social care and transport across the whole area (county). District, borough or city councils then deliver other services, including housing, council tax services and rubbish collection. District, borough or city councils deliver services to a smaller geographical area than a county council, so there may be a number of district, borough or city councils in one county.

Unitary or 'one-tier' areas

A 'one-tier' authority delivers all of the local authority services in a given area. One-tier authorities may be called unitary authorities, metropolitan boroughs or London boroughs.

Local public health teams are currently based in either county councils (upper tier) or unitary authorities. This means that they are often co-located with adult and children's services, which is useful for partnership working on service interventions. However, in two-tier areas, this means that local public health teams need to ensure there is close partnership working with district or borough councils as they are responsible for services such as housing, environmental health, planning, etc., which can have a big impact on the prevention of ill health and on improving the wider areas (determinants) that can influence health.

Roles and career opportunities

There is a wide range of roles and career opportunities within local authorities and generally there is no one set career path, although opportunities to develop professional careers in specialist areas such as housing, environmental health and social care do exist. For example, information about specialising in environmental health can be found earlier in this book and on the Chartered Institute of Environmental Health's website.[2] For those wishing to pursue a career in local government, a national graduate management development programme is available, which offers one way to do so. This is a two-year programme for graduates, during which projects are undertaken in a range of council departments. Some individual councils also run their own management programmes, details of which are usually available on individual councils' websites. Such programmes offer an opportunity to gain experience of the huge variety of different roles performed by a local authority. Such experience would be ideal preparation for a career in public health.

There are also many other roles in local authorities that can be applied for directly. This could include roles within a public health team in a local authority. However, roles within many other local authority teams may also be relevant to public health. In some local areas, local authority services may be outsourced to other organisations. For example, while housing, which has an important impact on people's health and wellbeing, is a local authority responsibility, in many areas local authority housing is managed by organisations called housing associations (or other similar organisations). Individuals who work for such organisations are not local authority employees, but they have an important role in addressing housing needs, and in neighbourhood and community development, which are important areas relating to public health. Further information about housing associations can be found on the National Housing Federation website.[3]

Similarly, different models exist in local areas for the provision of leisure and culture services (e.g. parks, sports facilities, etc.). Such services may be delivered by local authority staff, by trusts or by multiple providers contracted to deliver services.

Further information about culture and leisure can be found on the Chief Cultural and Leisure Officers' Association (CLOA) website.[4] Many of the skills and experience developed in such teams are likely to be useful in a future public health career.

Traditionally, much public health in local authorities has focused on health improvement. This is one of the key areas of public health in local authorities with positions additionally available in health protection, public health intelligence and health and social care quality. The following is a sample of job titles in the local authority public health team:

- Health and Wellbeing Project Officer
- Health Improvement Facilitator
- Health Intelligence Analyst
- Health, Wellbeing and Social Improvement Officer
- Health Policy Analyst.

Useful skills for working in a local authority

Some of the skills that may be useful to develop while working in a local authority on public health issues include the following.

Partnership working skills

Partnership working skills are important in local government, as many of the roles involve working with other organisations (public or private sector) or with the local community directly. An understanding of partners' perspectives and good communication and negotiation skills are really useful when working with other organisations.

Project management

Many public health projects in local authorities are complex, long-term projects involving many different organisations. Good project management skills can help to keep projects on track. Some councils offer internal project management training to staff, or external qualifications may be available (e.g. PRINCE II).

Report writing/analytical skills

Being able to write clear and concise reports is an important skill, as formal reports are required as part of decision-making processes in local government. Being able to communicate information to a wide range of audiences, including the public and people who are not health professionals, is also important. Basic numeracy (being comfortable with numbers) is helpful and this can be supplemented by additional training in statistical techniques.

Political awareness

As council decisions are made by elected councillors, it is useful to have a good understanding of the local political situation. This could include understanding the political make-up locally (e.g. how many councillors belong to each political party) and what the local and national position of different political parties is on public health issues. Understanding the historical context of an area may also be useful to understand activities of lobby groups, patient groups and other organisations that can support or differ from political decisions made by the local authority that affect public health.

Evidence-based practice

Understanding the evidence base behind a public health issue is an important skill, which can include identifying the strengths and limitations of evidence and providing an independent analysis, considering available evidence and research.

Achievements

There are many examples of achievements that local authorities have made in improving public health. One example is the Suffolk 'Warm homes, healthy people' project. This aimed to address winter deaths and fuel poverty as well as to reduce carbon emissions. It was a partnership project involving adult and community services (from the county council), environmental services (from the district and borough councils) and a host of voluntary and community sector partners. Public health teams were involved to support the partnership and to facilitate links with healthcare providers in order to generate referrals into the programme. The project enabled GPs, nurses, hospital discharge teams, children's centres and other teams to refer vulnerable clients. These clients were then able to receive direct payments to subsidise fuel bills, as well as home improvements such as loft and cavity wall insulation, boiler services, repairs or replacements and temporary heaters.

As part of a local authority team, it may be possible to apply for grants and awards, including local, national and international funding – for example, European Union funding – and to collaborate with others. After a successful public health project you may be asked to present the project at a conference. Presenting at conferences is a useful public health skill and proactively seeking these opportunities provides a good way of developing presentation skills.

Constraints and challenges

Financial challenges across the whole of the public sector mean that solutions to public health issues in local authority settings may need to be more creative to enable issues to be tackled despite financial constraints. Increasingly, opportunities are being developed for health and social care services to work together more closely and more efficiently – in an integrated way – which may involve closer sharing of information and resources.

How to get going

Some of the links below may be useful in finding out what roles and opportunities are available in local authorities.

- Local government jobs website: www.lgjobs.com/
- National Graduate Development Programme: www.ngdp.org.uk/
- Individual council websites
- Health Service Journal: www.hsj.co.uk/
- Leisure opportunities: www.leisureopportunities.co.uk/
- County Sports Partnerships: www.cspnetwork.org/en/recruitment/?s=o57WpEx5k 5XbkrLNT

Notes

1 Primary care groups and subsequently primary care trusts were introduced by the Labour government from 1999 as the main commissioners of healthcare.
2 Chartered Institute of Environmental Health. Available at: www.cieh.org.
3 National Housing Federation. Available at: www.housing.org.uk.
4 CLOA (Chief Cultural & Leisure Officers Association). Available at: www.cloa.org.uk.

Reference

Campbell, F. (ed.) *The social determinants of health and the role of local government.* London: IDeA, 2010.

8 National Health Service

Frances Fairman

Introduction to this setting

The National Health Service (NHS) is one of the largest organisations in the world and operates to common principles and nationwide pay scales. It is accountable via the Department of Health to central government and operates via annual funding from parliament. The NHS structures are different in each UK country (see the introductory part of this book), so health policy varies slightly from country to country. Public health practitioners may be employed in any NHS organisation, although in practice are most likely to be found in dedicated public health bodies, in commissioning agencies and in provider hospitals or other institutional and community-based providers of healthcare. Note that broadly similar roles may have quite different job titles.

EXAMPLE OF PUBLIC HEALTH PRACTITIONER ROLES IN THIS SETTING

The contributor presents what it means to work within the health service to ensure that commissioned care is based on the best available evidence of effectiveness and is affordable.

Frances Fairman, Clinical Effectiveness Manager

What is the job of 'clinical effectiveness manager' about?

The 'clinical effectiveness' function is rooted in 'evidence-based medicine'. It involves assessing evidence of the clinical effectiveness and cost-effectiveness of treatments and services, and presenting the findings ('best practice') as policies, guidelines or care pathways for the purpose of improving population health and wellbeing.

The publicly funded NHS, social care and public health services need the skills and knowledge of clinical effectiveness managers in order to ensure that high quality health services are provided, and it is for this reason that support for the clinical effectiveness function is enshrined in legislation. The NHS Constitution[1] gives patients a number of rights, including:

- the right to expect local decisions on funding of drugs and treatments to be made rationally following a proper consideration of the evidence; and
- the right to expect NHS organisations to monitor, and make efforts to improve, the quality of healthcare they commission or provide.

Providers and commissioners of health and social care must comply with the NHS Constitution, but there are other reasons why the clinical effectiveness function is needed:

- Much information is available to patients and the public about health treatments – through the Internet, on TV programmes and through social networking – resulting in increasing demand and higher expectations of the NHS.
- New – and generally more costly – treatments are continuously being introduced as a result of medical research and innovation in the healthcare industries.
- Public services 'need to do more with less', especially at times of economic downturn, when health and social care services must maintain or enhance services despite a real-terms reduction in government funding.

In this environment, the role of clinical effectiveness manager is one of the most interesting, challenging and rewarding jobs in public health. It is interesting because:

- it involves working at the leading edge of medicine and health service design, in liaison with researchers and innovators;
- it involves working with patients and the public as well as a wide range of organisations and individuals – hospital doctors, GPs, nurses and other clinicians, public health and local authorities, NHS healthcare commissioners and managers, researchers, medical librarians, the health service industries, health charities, politicians, the media and legal services;
- the function contributes to many kinds of projects – simple and complex, across all areas of health and social care, in both strategic and operational capacities – and no week is the same.

It is challenging because:

- the information and evidence needed is not always available or reliable;
- even if clinical evidence is available, it might be conflicting or not give clear answers, so sometimes difficult decisions have to be made;
- implementing the recommendations of the clinical effectiveness manager usually requires change, and changing the behaviour of organisations and individuals can be complex and time-consuming.

It is rewarding because:

- the clinical effectiveness role gives opportunities to influence policy and practice in the NHS and social care at a local, regional and national level;
- evaluation, clinical audit and patient feedback mechanisms show the impact of the clinical effectiveness manager's work;
- the clinical effectiveness manager has opportunities for on-going learning, development and career progression.

What does a clinical effectiveness manager do?

The role will vary according to the structure they work in, but most clinical effectiveness managers are responsible for the day-to-day operational management and strategic planning of an extensive programme of work, including developing and implementing clinical commissioning policies and service redesign projects that will result in better quality of care and provide best value for the population they serve.

To deliver their objectives, a clinical effectiveness manager needs information about what is happening across their local health system. For example, they need to know how healthy the population is compared with other areas, whether there are variations in quality of healthcare between different hospitals and services, and how much money is being spent. The clinical effectiveness manager's colleagues in the public health team will provide information about health inequalities and the likely health needs of the local population. There are a number of national and regional data sources that the clinical effectiveness manager can tap into to see where local services might not be delivering the quality and type of care needed. 'Horizon scanning' is very important – clinical effectiveness managers need to identify new treatments in the pipeline, or new national standards or policies that should be implemented locally, in order to plan future health services.

Where opportunities for improvement are identified, the clinical effectiveness manager may work alone or as a member of a project team to bring about the changes needed. Their role might be to establish whether a specific treatment is clinically effective, or which of a number of treatment options works best and is the most affordable for the NHS locally. Or the clinical effectiveness manager might be asked to assess the evidence for different models of healthcare provision – for example, whether patients with long-term conditions should be reviewed regularly in a hospital setting, or whether 'telehealth' is as effective. A clinical effectiveness manager may also support public health by investigating whether programmes to prevent ill health are effective and represent the best value – for example, weight-loss programmes that are intended to prevent the health problems associated with obesity.

In particular, the function of the clinical effectiveness manager is to help reduce health inequalities – inequalities that may arise because of insufficient services available to some patient groups (e.g. if the make-up of the local population includes people originally from South Asia, then enhanced diabetic services may be needed as the incidence of the disease is higher in this population group); because of variations in the treatment offered by different healthcare providers (e.g. because of clinicians' research interests); or because of access issues (e.g. elderly people without means of transport or rural location). The clinical effectiveness manager will work with commissioners of healthcare not only to ensure that clinically effective and cost-effective treatments are available, but that services are prioritised or enhanced to ensure they reach patient groups with the greatest unmet needs.

Because a clinical effectiveness manager seeks to ensure that the NHS invests in treatments and services that work and also give value for money, they are also involved in disinvesting from less effective services. This area of work can be particularly challenging and complex, especially where clinicians and patients value a service, and health systems to deliver it are well established. Nevertheless, it is essential that resources are used to achieve the greatest health benefits, and the clinical effectiveness manager may need to present evidence to public board meetings, or be involved in public consultation and engagement exercises to help to justify the difficult decisions being made.

Sometimes clinicians will request funding for a treatment for an individual patient that is not normally provided by the NHS. For example, a clinician may want to treat a rare condition with a drug that is not licensed for that particular use. In these instances, a clinical effectiveness manager will look at all available evidence in the context of the individual patient's specific health problem and report the findings to a decision-making panel. Rarely, individual patients will appeal against funding decisions made by their local NHS by requesting a judicial review. The work of the clinical effectiveness manager will be under scrutiny in such court cases, as the judge will require documented proof that the funding decision had been made following due process and consideration of the relevant clinical evidence.

In order to achieve their objectives, a clinical effectiveness manager will seek to develop and maintain a culture of continuous evidence-based improvement in their organisation. They will also look for opportunities to raise awareness and promote learning about clinical effectiveness. The latter may include talks to patient groups, teaching students, as well as media releases on topical issues.

What work settings and career opportunities are there for clinical effectiveness managers?

The restructuring of the NHS in England in 2013 means that there are new opportunities for clinical effectiveness managers to work in local, regional and national settings.

In England, local roles are available in GP-led Clinical Commissioning Groups (CCGs) and in public health teams based in local authorities. Clinical Commissioning Groups[2] will need the skills of clinical effectiveness managers to help them develop evidence-based tools to commission high quality care from their local healthcare providers. These tools may include local commissioning policies; evidence-based guidelines that specify the treatments that should be provided by their local hospitals or community services; plans for disinvesting from less effective treatments, and the introduction of new and more effective treatments; and dealing with individual requests for treatments that are not normally funded.

Public health teams based in local authorities[3] need the skills of clinical effectiveness managers to support decision-making about priorities for health and social care services for the local population. This includes identifying the populations with the greatest healthcare needs and advising on the most clinically and cost-effective treatments and services to reduce health inequalities. Public health teams may also need their clinical effectiveness managers to provide advice to their local CCGs on areas where there is potential for disinvestment or to enable the relative value of competing demands to be assessed. Clinical effectiveness managers may also need to advise on the local impact of new national guidance, such as that from NICE (the National Institute of Health and Care Excellence), and other new drugs/technologies and innovations within the local health economy, and assist with prioritisation. Where finances are tight, the clinical effectiveness manager contributes to ensuring that evidence is used to help make correct decisions about how resources are appropriately prioritised towards those with the greatest needs and that services provide good value for money.

Opportunities also exist at regional level in the newly formed Commissioning Support Units,[4] which may be contracted to provide 'clinical effectiveness' functions for groups of Clinical Commissioning Groups. In this setting, the clinical effectiveness manager will be able to influence the implementation of evidence-based policies across a wider geographical area and with several providers of health and social care. A regional role requires the clinical effectiveness manager to work across a number of 'stakeholder' organisations and work strategically to make system-wide changes happen.

National opportunities for clinical effectiveness managers will be available in NHS England and in Public Health England. The NHS Commissioning Board (known as NHS England) directly commissions 'specialised services' across England as a whole. Specialised health services are those required to treat people with rare health conditions where there are few clinicians with the expertise and knowledge to treat them. Many long-term conditions that affect children, and children's surgery, come under the umbrella of specialised commissioning. This area of evidence-based medicine can be particularly interesting and challenging for clinical effectiveness managers as there is generally a lack of published evidence to support decision-making.

As well as these opportunities in England, there are comparable roles in NHS Scotland, Wales and Northern Ireland within their own health service structures.

Once obtained, the skills of the clinical effectiveness manager can be transferred to healthcare research or systematic reviewer roles in the public or independent sectors. In the future, large hospital trusts may also recognise the need for the clinical effectiveness manager's skills to help them with the introduction of innovations and the development of evidence-based business cases.

What knowledge and skills do you need to be a clinical effectiveness manager?

The description of the tasks of the clinical effectiveness manager above highlight the wide range of public health skills and knowledge needed for the role. Some of these can be obtained through formal training courses but many of the competences required for the role can be obtained through on-the-job training and development.

Clinical effectiveness managers may have a clinical background (e.g. pharmacist or nurse training) but this is not essential. Clinical effectiveness managers are usually educated to degree level or have equivalent work experience. Some senior roles may require a Master's qualification (e.g. in public health, health care management or health economics).

Clinical effectiveness managers need an understanding of epidemiology, statistics, health economics and healthcare evaluation. In particular, they should have a practical knowledge of change management to enable them to embed service improvement and evidence-based clinical practice. Some of these skills can be learned through training courses; others may be gained through work experience.

It is also important to have a good understanding of national health and social care policies and standards, as well as local issues and priorities, from both the 'commissioner' and 'healthcare provider' perspectives. This knowledge of the (often complex) political and social environment is needed as the work of the clinical effectiveness manager should be incorporated into strategic plans, be realistic, and have the endorsement of stakeholders. Clinical effectiveness managers also need to be aware of the legislation that applies to the health and social care services.

Research, analytical and numerical skills are essential requirements for a clinical effectiveness manager. The technical and analytical skills required include the ability to write 'search strategies', undertake literature searches of medical databases and other resources, and 'critically appraise' research articles to distil and summarise the evidence of clinical and cost-effectiveness that they contain. These skills can be developed through attendance on short training courses (e.g. medical statistics and basic health economics; literature searching skills are often taught by healthcare librarians in hospitals and research centres), but clinical effectiveness managers need to underpin this with a meticulous and systematic approach to their work.

Communication skills are very important. Clinical effectiveness managers have to be able to present complex information and ideas in ways that enable different audiences to understand it. The audiences might be board members, patient groups, public meetings, individuals who don't have English as their first language, clinicians and politicians. Clinical effectiveness managers use evidence and information to bring about change and therefore need to be able to speak effectively at meetings, write papers and reports, and deliver presentations. In tandem with this, clinical effectiveness managers must quickly establish effective working relationships across organisational and professional boundaries, and facilitate team work. *Project management* training is very useful in this respect, as are the leadership skills to motivate colleagues and deliver projects to time and within budget.

Clinical effectiveness managers need to keep up to date with new developments in health and social care – being able to read quickly helps.

Examples of instances where the work of a clinical effectiveness manager has made a difference

Stopping people having surgery unnecessarily

There is always a risk to health from surgery, especially if a general anaesthetic is required. Clinical effectiveness managers are particularly focused on ensuring that only those patients who will benefit from a treatment are offered it, and a review of the benefits of a surgical intervention is always accompanied by an analysis of the possible harms or adverse effects. As well as a review of the clinical and cost-effectiveness, this type of project involves liaison with surgeons, GPs and patient groups to agree clinical criteria for surgery. Clinical criteria for treatments are usually published in the form of policy statements or referral guidelines. NHS commissioning organisations that have these types of policies in place are able to control demand for treatments and manage the pressure on health services by ensuring that the people likely to gain the greatest benefit are prioritised for treatment.

Patient decision aids

It is important that patients are given accurate information about the effect that treatments might have on their future function and quality of life so that they can give informed consent. 'Decision aids' are particularly helpful for patients who might have a choice of types of surgery (e.g. 'open' or 'laparoscopic') or drug treatments, and can form the basis for discussions between the patient and their doctor when the patient is making their treatment choice.

A clinical effectiveness manager developed evidence-based patient decision aids for hip and knee replacement surgery, which specified the likely benefits and harms, both short and long term, and enabled individuals to assess whether joint replacement surgery was right for them.

Resource allocation and priority setting

A clinical effectiveness manager helped an ambulance service to decide how best to deploy its ambulance teams by undertaking an evidence review of the effectiveness of 'Community First Responders' (CFRs). CFRs are trained members of a local population – usually living in villages or remote locations – who provide initial assessment and first aid in health emergencies. By augmenting the ambulance service in rural areas, CFRs may avoid the need for an emergency ambulance to take a patient to hospital or may 'buy time' before an ambulance arrives. The evidence review helped the ambulance service and commissioners decide whether to invest in CFRs or look for alternative models for the delivery of emergency care in less accessible areas.

Public health prevention programmes

In trying to decide how to allocate its stretched resources, a local authority requested a review of the evidence of the effectiveness of roadside speed cameras in reducing death and injury on the roads to see if they represented value for money. An evidence appraisal by the clinical effectiveness manager was used to gain agreement to maintain the speed cameras in specific 'black spots'.

Service redesign

The issue of the rationalisation of hospital services is highly political. Hospital trusts commonly operate over a number of sites and, for efficiency, safety and cost-saving reasons, may wish to close a local hospital. In one instance a trust was required by the government to keep a district hospital open, and the hospital asked the clinical effectiveness manager to identify and review national and international evidence to help them decide which clinical services would be viable for a small, rural hospital. The majority of doctors, nurses and management staff affected were resistant to the resultant changes but the use of evidence helped move the negotiations forward.

Further information on the role of clinical effectiveness manager

You can find out more by looking at the websites listed below, which provide information about various aspects of 'evidence-based healthcare' and improving public health. If you think it could be the career for you, you will need to have a degree and be willing to undertake further training and development as you progress.

Notes

1 www.nhs.uk/choiceintheNHS/Rightsandpledges/NHSConstitution/Pages/Overview.aspx
2 Clinical Commissioning Groups (CCGs) from April 2013 are responsible for commissioning 60 per cent of secondary care in England.
3 Under the Health and Social Care Act 2012, upper tier local authorities are charged under their additional public health responsibilities with providing public health advice to the NHS.
4 Commissioning Support Units created under the coalition government reforms as part of NHS England to provide contracting and commissioning support to CCGs.

Suggested follow-up references

Bad Science by Ben Goldacre: www.badscience.net/
Cochrane Collaboration: www.cochrane.org/
The Cochrane Library: www.thecochranelibrary.com/view/0/index.html
The Campbell Collaboration: www.campbellcollaboration.org/
NHS Evidence: www.evidence.nhs.uk/
NICE (National Institute for Health and Care Excellence): www.nice.org.uk/ and particu-
    larly, 'About NICE': www.nice.org.uk/aboutnice/about_nice.jsp
Public Health Intelligence: www.phe.org.uk
'Right Care' and the NHS Atlas of Variation: www.rightcare.nhs.uk/index.php/nhs-atlas/

9 Health policy settings

Mohit Sharma

Introduction to this setting

Public health practitioners working on health policy can be based in a range of different settings, including civil service and governmental organisations. Those aiming to influence policy-making are often employed by the third sector – that is, organisations that are not-for-profit and non-governmental lobbying groups (in contrast to the private and public sectors) – and some policy analysts work within academic institutions.

EXAMPLE OF PUBLIC HEALTH PRACTITIONER ROLES IN THIS SETTING

The following contribution looks at the opportunities to influence health policy within national settings, from a public health practitioner in training for a career as a consultant in public health, including his personal experience and career journey.

Mohit Sharma, Specialty Registrar in Public Health: National Health Policy

Introduction

Public health makes a very valuable contribution to national policy on health and the wider determinants of health, the things that enable us to live our lives to their full potential and reduce our chances of ill health. Training in public health provides many opportunities to contribute to national policy development and this chapter gives a personal perspective on the opportunities gained during specialist training in public health.

What is policy?

In the broadest sense, policy refers to a general principle or rule to guide action. This is usually needed when decisions need to be made about complex issues or where consistency in decision-making is required. These principles or rules may be applicable to governments, public or private organisations, or to groups and individuals. At the national level, policy guides the action of a broad range of organisations to address particular ends such as addressing inequalities or ensuring the provision of treatments to all those who may benefit from them. Developing policy requires the development and use of a sound evidence base, but this in itself is not sufficient as policy is influenced by the political context and this needs to be understood and managed. To be effective in delivering the intent, there needs to be planning in place from the outset about the implementation of the policy. There are many influences on the development of policy from those with expertise in the subject areas, those affected by the policy recommendations and those with the responsibility for implementation. All of these various groups, or stakeholders, should be involved in the development of the policy through consultation at all stages of policy-making.

Public health specialists and practitioners have skills in the development, understanding and use of evidence, expert understanding of health systems, and understanding and managing the political context of policy development and implementation. This makes public health specialists well placed to inform the development of policy at all stages.

How does national policy influence health?

In the UK, national policy is the context within which health and other relevant services are developed and delivered. National policy, informed by evidence, highlights the areas that need to be priorities for health services and other services that impact on people's health. Policy decisions impact, for example, on the resources available to services locally, impacting on patients who need those services. National policy also helps to address broader issues that must be addressed collectively by society, such as the need to reduce health inequalities (the disparity in health outcomes between groups in society).

English Department of Health

The Department of Health is the leading government department in each country responsible for health and has a very important role in setting policy. Health services are directly responsible to the Department of Health and are shaped by national policy from the Department of Health. Other government departments are responsible for policy in their areas such as the economy, transport and welfare, and these policies also have an influence on the health of people. So the Department of Health also seeks to influence the policies of other government departments where they influence the health of the population.

The Department of Health employs people from a range of backgrounds, including public health specialists, the career civil service, those from medical and from non-medical backgrounds. Often the people involved may have specific expertise to contribute to the policy process, such as specialist clinicians or patients who have had the condition, and their involvement may be for short periods. As a consequence, policy teams can be fluid with new people joining and others leaving within short periods of time. Working in this situation demands rapidly developing an appreciation of the perspectives and knowledge of others, and the ability to communicate ideas clearly to all. The work can be intense and have very tight timescales requiring flexibility and an ability to work under pressure.

Much of the work in policy development requires negotiating and influencing skills to ensure that the aims of the policy can be met to the satisfaction of all partners and this is a skill that requires practice to develop, but is essential to influence policy. All policy development has a political context that must be understood and managed. This is particularly true in a government department where the minister responsible for directing policy has to be briefed on the developing policy from time to time.

More broadly, there are opportunities in all aspects of policy work from development and implementation to evaluation, though the specific areas will vary with the team and the stage of policy development at any time. Most valuable is the opportunity to work with many national leaders.

Training in public health in the Department of Health

Training to be a specialist in public health in the Department of Health provides the opportunity to learn about the development, implementation and impact of policies. There is a wide range of work that can be undertaken with different teams in the department and can address almost all of the skills that trainees need to develop. In particular, the department is a good place to work for developing the skills for working with colleagues from diverse backgrounds, developing negotiating and influencing skills, developing leadership skills, and working on all aspects of policy development, implementation and evaluation. Working in the Department of Health is a very good opportunity to observe and understand the political influences in the development of national policy and to observe national leaders in action and learn from them. For a trainee it was very instructive to observe the leadership styles of different national leaders, to understand the differences in their leadership styles, and then to reflect on what I could apply to develop my leadership style.

National Institute for Health and Care Excellence

The National Institute for Health and Care Excellence (NICE) is a non-departmental public body (an 'arm's-length body') responsible for providing national guidance on the promotion of good health, and the prevention and treatment of ill health. NICE guidance is mainly applicable to the NHS, healthcare organisations and their users, though NICE is now responsible for producing guidance for social care as well. Its broader guidance on the promotion of good health and prevention is of interest to health services, local authorities, independent and voluntary sectors. The guidance produced by NICE ranges from appraisals of single technologies (such as new drugs) to guidance on medical devices and clinical guidelines for diagnosis and management of particular conditions (such as stroke or diabetes). Guidance from technology appraisals *must* be implemented by the NHS while clinical guidelines recommend best practice that the NHS should deliver and that patients can expect.

Clinical guidelines are based on evidence of what works best for patients and are formed by independent advisory committees with input from experts (clinicians and health service managers), and patients and lay representatives. Guidelines are developed with equity and social values in mind; as for policy development, there is wide consultation with those affected by the guidelines, including the public.

NICE guidance informs clinicians and patients about the most effective ways to diagnose, treat and prevent disease and ill health that are also best value for money. The guidance allows health services managers, local authorities, charities and anyone with a responsibility for commissioning or providing healthcare to provide the best services for patients. As such, NICE guidance has an influence on patients across the country in ensuring that the services that they need are consistently available and provide the treatments that have been shown to work.

My experience in working at a national level on policy affecting health

I started my career with graduation in medicine and then specialisation in surgery. Advances in treatment, changes in government priorities, and changes in the expectations and experiences of patients led to a change in working practices and the organisation of services in hospitals. It became apparent to me that my work, the working of the hospital and the wider health system were changing due to changes in national policy. This led me to think of the wide influence of policy on many and the limited influence that an individual doctor has on the population. I decided to develop my skills in order to influence policy decisions, and as public health training provides an understanding of how policy is developed and applied, I joined the public health training scheme.

On the public health training scheme I have worked with the Department of Health and with NICE, both national organisations with a major role in the development of national policy. My work with the Department of Health was a placement with the Local Public Health Systems team within the Public Health England Transition Team, involved in the transition to Public Health England, the new national public health agency, and the transition of public health to local government. My work with NICE was as a NICE scholar, conducting a project with support from NICE and with the opportunity to observe the working of NICE committees to develop an understanding of the work of NICE.

Training opportunities with NICE

NICE is described as a 'national treasure' for public health training[1] so that placements with NICE are possible for public health trainees from anywhere in the UK. Clinical trainees also have opportunities to work with NICE. There may in addition be development opportunities with NICE for people from other backgrounds.

The skills required for working with NICE

The skills needed to work on the development of guidance require an understanding of evidence, an ability to work with a range of people with different expertise, and an ability to seek the views of others and have regard to social values. This would usually mean having a background in health research or in clinical medicine with expertise of a specific area (such as cardiology or diabetes); or public health expertise with the skills of understanding research, the purpose, principles and methods of guidance production; and working with others in the development of guidelines or policy. More details on the specific skills needed for particular roles are available from NICE.

How to get involved

Meetings of NICE advisory committees are held in public and can be observed. Further involvement in developing the guidance is possible for lay people, patients or carers, and for professionals. Professionals need to have either clinical expertise, health services management expertise or health research expertise. Information on the work of NICE, and on opportunities for working with NICE is available on the NICE website.

Other national policy opportunities

The Department of Health and NICE are two of a number of different organisations that have an important influence on national health policy. There are a range of other organisations where it is possible to gain national policy experience, including medical royal colleges, medical and public health charities (such as the British Heart Foundation and Cancer Research UK) and think tanks (such as the Nuffield Trust and King's Fund) who are all involved in shaping and influencing national policy.

Skills needed for working on national policy to influence health

The skills needed in all of these organisations are similar, requiring an understanding of evidence, and an ability to work with, and seek the views of others in developing solutions that are shown to work and best address the needs of patients. The skills can be gained through medical training and public health training or through work as a practitioner in the health service. Public health training develops skills in all aspects of evidence interpretation and policy development. Medical training with development of specific expertise in a particular area will be valuable for policy in that area of clinical care. Experience in health research also helps to develop some of the skills required for policy development, particularly the understanding and application of evidence. Civil service training develops skills in policy development across government departments, including the Department of Health.

What can be gained from working with national policy-oriented organisations?

Developing policy requires an application of the evidence to ensure that the chosen options are those that work best for patients. This evidence of what works needs to be applied in the political context of the policy formulation and both of these are very relevant to the final policy developed. So while NICE guidance relies more on the evidence base, though it is developed in a political context, broader health policy developed by the Department of Health is much more reflective of the political context, though it is also largely based on evidence where available. Having exposure to these different contexts of policy development allows one the opportunity to understand the political influence on policy that shapes the environments within which we work and live.

The organisations that develop national policy involve a wide range of national leaders, and having the opportunity to observe them in action is invaluable in understanding leadership styles to develop my leadership skills. Working on development, implementation and evaluation of national policy is an excellent opportunity to understand the processes and complexities of the task, and to then be able to develop the ability to manage the challenges and conflicts in the process.

Summary

Policy development is carried out by a range of organisations nationally and requires a broad-based set of skills with understanding of evidence and an understanding of the political context in which the policy is being developed. These skills can be gained in different ways, including public health training, health research and the civil service. However, policy development is not the sole preserve of the 'expert' and there are opportunities for lay persons to influence this as well, through NICE and other national organisations. Ultimately, national policy influences the things that enable us all to live our lives to their full potential and reduce our chances of ill health: contributing to this is very rewarding.

Note

1 Status conferred by the UK Faculty of Public Health for placements for trainees where very specific skills can be acquired.

References

Department of Health, London. Available at: www.gov.uk/government/topics/public-health. Accessed 22 June 2014.

Department of Health, London. Available at: www.gov.uk/government/publications/the-health-and-care-system-explained. Accessed 22 June 2014.

National Institute for Health and Care Excellence (NICE). Available at: www.nice.org.uk/. Accessed 22 June 2014.

Nuffield Trust. Available at: www.nuffieldtrust.org.uk/about/what-we-do. Accessed 22 June 2014.

Public Health England. Available at: www.gov.uk/government/organisations/public-health-england. Accessed 22 June 2014.

Sim, F. and McKee, M. *Issues in Public Health*. 2nd edn, Open University Press, 2013.

World Health Organization. Available at: www.who.int/topics/health_policy/en/. Accessed 22 June 2014.

International and global health

Jenny Amery; Manpreet Singh; Manuelle Hurwitz

Introduction to this setting

Public health practitioners may work for a number of different agencies in delivering public health and humanitarian services around the world. These can be governmental, non-governmental organisations or charitable institutions. Some of the most common agencies are listed on the UK Public Health Careers website (www.phorcast.org.uk) – such as Médecins Sans Frontières, Merlin, Oxfam, Health-Eu and also where to go for further information).

EXAMPLES OF PUBLIC HEALTH PRACTITIONER ROLES IN THIS SETTING

The three contributors in this chapter provide very different perspectives on what it means to work in international public health at different points in your career. Two outline how you can contribute in senior and junior roles and the third presents a personal perspective.

Jenny Amery, DFID: a career in international public health

Introduction

According to family folklore, at the age of five, sitting on my maternal grandmother's knee, I announced 'when I grow up I am going to work in Africa'. My grandparents had lived and worked in India and in their sitting room in Somerset, a series of brass elephants marched across the mantelpiece, and there was a fading and rather mysterious painting of the Taj Mahal on the wall. I have actually worked mostly in Latin America and Asia, rather than Africa, but every international public health practitioner will have a story to tell.

Working and living in low-resource communities

I joined a workcamp to help build a school in East Africa in my summer break while a medical student, which opened my eyes to many things. My working years overseas have been mostly in poor communities in Latin America and India. These have undoubtedly been among my most formative professional experiences. After qualifying as a doctor and working in child health and obstetrics, I went with a volunteer organisation to live and work with the Amuesha Indians in the Peruvian Amazon rainforest, to deliver primary care services in a river-based network and train community health workers. Those were politically turbulent times, and after eighteen months I moved to a national NGO to help develop child health and nutrition services with impoverished shanty-town dwellers in Chimbote, the port where cholera was later reintroduced to Peru and to the Americas after decades free of the disease. I then went on to work for two years on women's health in shanty towns in Chile under the dictatorship of Augusto Pinochet.

I have worked for the UK government's Department for International Development (DFID) since 1999, and lived in Delhi for three years during that time, working in some of the poorest communities in that vast country of over one billion people. I have worked with many remarkable individuals and organisations across the world, formulating policy; designing, implementing and reviewing programmes; finding, assessing and applying evidence in practice; and leading the expanding cadre of DFID health professionals worldwide, now numbering over seventy. I like to think that something of my grandmother's spirit of concern, commitment and adventure has stayed with me.

What is international public health about?

International public health is about working with individuals, authorities, countries, across borders and sometimes across the globe, to improve the health of populations, and often focusing on the needs of the poorest and those most at risk. As with all public health approaches, it involves analysis of the problem, formulation and testing of solutions, making decisions, influencing others, securing funds, ensuring systems to monitor progress and impact, seeking views from many quarters and sticking with commitments for the long haul – and learning lessons.

Health is recognised, although not always protected, as a basic human right. It is both a result of and contributor to poverty reduction, and is linked to macroeconomic growth. There is currently a welcome consensus and global commitment (but not yet achieved) led by the World Health Organization, to universal access to essential health services (protection, prevention, treatment and care). Good health and wellbeing require a lot more than health services – clearly demonstrated by the marked falls in death rates from the introduction of safe drinking water, sanitation, better housing, improved nutrition and clean air in nineteenth-century Britain. However, effective services are a key part of the solution. Prominence has been given recently in the UK and globally to the social determinants of health, including education, personal safety, women's empowerment, water sanitation and hygiene (WASH), nutrition, and many others.

Working in public health requires a clear vision of what you are aiming for and commitment for the long term, with milestones on the way and flexibility in the 'how' of achieving them. There are relatively few quick successes and they may be short-lived.

Despite impressive progress globally, many of the health challenges in the very poor communities where I worked in the 1980s are still relevant. For example, improving the nutrition of young women pre-pregnancy; ensuring early and exclusive breast feeding; adequate micronutrients; access to nutritious food (even when it is plentiful) for women and girls; agricultural policies that lead to better nutrition rather than just higher crop yields; ensuring children are vaccinated and protected against preventable diseases, and many more. While working as a volunteer doctor in Peru I realised that however hard I worked to save the lives of individual children, they would keep falling ill until the root causes of their illness and poverty were addressed. I wrote a book on the causes and solutions to the unacceptably high child deaths and rates of disease in that country, co-authored a book on infant feeding and moved gradually from clinical work to training, action-research, advocacy and collaborative work with the local social justice commission. I learned a huge amount from local political and social scientists, activists and community leaders. Peru is one of the countries where there has been significant progress on nutrition policy and child health outcomes.

On return from overseas, I entered the UK NHS five-year public health training programme, and completed the Faculty (of Public Health) exams. This gave me a solid scientific grounding, supervised opportunities to apply it in different settings, some media skills, an awareness of my own limitations and the importance of working with, training and supporting others. I learned how important good team-working is to achieving public health impact – and the need to make public health issues everyone's business!

How has international public health made a difference?

There has been huge progress globally in the health of the poorest people. Child mortality in almost all African countries has fallen dramatically in the last thirty years; maternal deaths are at last falling, although the lifetime risk of dying in childbirth of one in sixteen for women in some parts of Africa and South Asia remains shockingly high and contrasts starkly with the very minimal risk in rich countries. Cases and deaths from malaria have been dramatically reduced in many of the worst affected countries. Other infectious diseases are close to elimination. Polio is now endemic in only three countries globally. In all of these examples, public health practitioners have played key roles in developing the evidence for effective action in low-resource or remote settings, mobilising the political commitment and funding, skilling-up professionals and communities (for example, ensuring grandmothers, partners and others know the key danger signs for a pregnant woman when she should seek care immediately), developing tools to measure progress and strategies when progress falters, and keeping up the momentum when fatigue threatens.

Much international public health effort is concerned with reducing the stark inequalities in health outcomes between social and economic quintiles, ethnic or religious groups, geographical regions, men and women. However, well-intentioned policies to provide services for the poorest do not always reach them, or may not be accessed by them even if they are geographically close, for reasons of cost, attitude and behaviours of staff, or cultural issues. I have learned how important it is to listen to what local people have to say about what they need, how their lives are constrained, what their priorities are.

The national and local public health leadership and capacity in many less developed countries are scarce, but growing. International public health support is often very important in disease outbreaks such as cholera or the Ebola virus, in emergencies and protracted political instability, but it is not without its limitations and risks of failure, particularly if done without taking adequate account of the political and power dynamics. Increasingly, and rightly, in many countries, the leadership is local, and international agencies are mandated to support local strategic priorities and work together to deliver these. It is important to avoid international staff duplicating some technical or geographical areas, poaching local staff and paying them inflated salaries, or ignoring issues they are not interested in – some of the poor practices that have grown up in the increasingly crowded field of health aid and which mean that much less is achieved for the resources put in.

It has taken decades to get child and intergenerational undernutrition into the global health development priorities. For too long nutrition has been everyone's and therefore no one's priority, in government, academia, the UN or international development agencies. Pot-bellied, wasted-limbed children in famines generate short-term relief funding, but there has been insufficient sustained effort to prevent the long-term damage to generations of children's lives from chronic undernutrition and stunting. In the otherwise influential Millennium Development Goals, undernutrition was obscured in the first goal by the focus on improving average incomes. However, that is changing. International public health leaders have used robust research for effective advocacy, including highlighting the glacial speed of the reduction of undernutrition, even in countries with sustained economic growth and overall food security. There has been remarkable progress in other economically growing countries (Brazil, for example). Longitudinal studies that follow undernourished children over time have highlighted its hugely negative impact on children's health, ability to learn, social development and skills, and earning potential. In some cases countries with rising GDP and wealth have been stirred into action. In India, I worked closely with officials in some of the poorest states to ensure cost-effective nutrition interventions were provided as a part of their health programmes. However, more action is needed beyond health interventions.

Sometimes a public health success is when something did not happen. For example, not having a cholera outbreak after disastrous flooding and contamination of water supplies in overcrowded shanty towns is a major triumph, but rarely makes headlines.

Working for a government department

Where I work, in the UK Department for International Development (DFID), all members of the multidisciplinary cadre of health professionals have strong public health competencies. We work in decentralised offices in some of the poorest countries in the world, with national governments, policy-makers, civil society groups and private-sector entities. We contribute, for example, to policies and programmes to improve maternal and child health, ensuring that all women have access to reproductive health services. We advocate policies on the sustainable financing of health services, and the prevention of catastrophic health payments that result in families selling their few assets and falling into poverty. We also advocate and fund clean water and sanitation as major contributors to better health. We work with partners to monitor implementation of policies, and to try to understand what is not working, as much as what is.

As staff of DFID we have privileged access to government ministers and officials, opinion leaders in universities, public and private services, think tanks and others. We have to know and stick to the facts, use hard evidence, and always prepare. If we voice an opinion, we state that it is only an opinion. We need to understand the politics and especially the power dynamics. It is also important to know your own limitations, and always know someone you can turn to when at the limits of your own knowledge or skills. Important although not always easy, is seeking feedback and learning from your mistakes.

Working in a government department requires adherence to the civil service values of integrity, honesty, objectivity and impartiality. If passionate advocacy is your mission, then it may not be the place for you.

Incoming governments may not wish to keep commitments made by the previous government, and often want to start their own initiatives, aspiring to show quick results. The challenge is to engage ministers on the basis of robust evidence. Politics is sometimes defined as the art of the possible. As a public health professional, it is vital to maintain your professional and personal values at all times.

Job and career opportunities

Health is increasingly seen by people inside and outside public health as a global security issue. Potential and actual new health threats spread across the world very fast – for example, the emergence of new diseases, such as HIV/AIDS in the 1980s, SARS in China in 2003, the on-going risk of pandemic flu, and the increasing resistance to modern antibiotics of the microorganisms responsible for tuberculosis, malaria and many other infectious diseases. The health of the population of every country is of importance globally, well beyond its borders. On cue, step up public health experts, to strengthen systems for early detection, identification of the emerging disease, evidence-based control measures, and more. The Royal Institute of International Affairs policy centre in London, better known as Chatham House, runs a programme on Global

Health Security. New opportunities for public health professionals are appearing around the world.

International public health job opportunities are many and changing. Working within an organisational structure is important in any setting, but particularly when working in a 'less developed' country. Understanding and addressing local priorities, listening to and learning from local practitioners, making efforts to follow and understand the power and political dynamics, are key to having a positive impact and minimising the risks of negative ones. What you do is often more powerful than what you say. There are opportunities in the multilateral agencies (World Health Organization (WHO), United Nations Children's Fund (UNICEF), United Nations Population Fund (UNFPA), United Nations Programme on HIV/AIDS (UNAIDS), World Bank and other development banks, European Commission). There are opportunities also in bilateral government agencies (e.g. the UK Department for International Development (DFID), in non-governmental organisations (NGOs) such as Save the Children, Oxfam, Médecins Sans Frontières (MSF), and many more; in university departments and other research organisations; in private foundations (Bill and Melinda Gates Foundation, Clinton Foundation, Wellcome Trust and more), and in private-sector organisations. Increasingly, these involve working in close partnership with national governments and agencies to strengthen their capacity and ensure the sustainability of work beyond the lifetime of externally funded projects.

International NGOs offer fascinating opportunities to work with some of the most marginalised communities, in humanitarian or development settings. There may be scope for people with knowledge and skills in public health, but relatively limited international experience. Language skills are a huge asset, and can be acquired through intense training. Learning in a setting where the language being learned is the dominant one, and you have to make an effort in every bus or marketplace encounter, is easily the most effective – and fun.

An issue of increasing concern not just to us as public health practitioners, but to the people on whose behalf we are working, is the accountability of international organisations and practitioners: accountability upwards to sovereign elected governments and to government funders for their money. Often forgotten and of crucial importance, however, is accountability to the people who are using services, and indirectly paying for them with their taxes and community contributions. In even the poorest countries, the greatest share of the health budget is from domestic funds, not international ones.

Public health-trained professionals bring a unique population perspective to health challenges. Some of us have been clinically trained and have worked at the front line delivering services to individuals. This gives privileged insight into the lives of people, often in great adversity. There is no substitute for this experience, and I would recommend that graduates in clinical professions take enough time to get 'front-line' experience before embarking on a public health career. Others will join international public health after studying or working in economics, geography, statistics, international relations and diplomacy, social policy or research, and many other disciplines and jobs.

Public health roles involve data, evidence and population numbers (instead of faces, names and life stories), policy choices, budget allocations and trade-offs. Of course, clinicians face these issues too, but their primary loyalty is to their individual patient. Public health practitioners are aiming for the greatest benefit for the population as well as benefits for individuals; maintaining intellectual and practical curiosity is crucial. What makes life in public health so interesting is the constant opportunity to ask why, and why not, and how best, and how not to, and to pursue the answers, and try to anticipate the unintended consequences. Day to day you can find yourself immersed in data analysis; talking to an on-line community of (professional) practice or an international conference; meeting community leaders, government ministers and officials, opposition leaders, health professionals; visiting rural (or urban) clinical services; worrying about your carbon footprint, and much more.

Manpreet Singh: working in international and global health as a public health practitioner

Working in global public health allows you to immerse yourself into new countries and cultures, to work with exceptional people from a broad range of professional backgrounds, and to constantly stretch yourself and work outside your comfort zone. Most importantly, working in international public health allows you to make a real difference to the lives of the poorest and most in-need people across the world. This chapter is an attempt to explain why we're enthusiastic about global public health, to explain the range of opportunities available for everyone and to outline next steps to take if you're interested in a career in global public health.

Description of the function

At its simplest level, as a global public health practitioner, you are working to improve the health of people across the world. Traditionally, this has been interpreted as the developing world, including sub-Saharan Africa, Central and South America, Eastern Europe and Central and South Asia. In many ways, separating global health from Western public health is a false split – many of the problems tackled are the same, including reducing inequalities in health, increasing access to health services for the poorest and helping tackle the root causes of ill health. As you will learn through the rest of this book, public health is all about looking at the bigger picture and developing systems to improve the health of people at a population level.

Roles

Jobs in global health are varied, with opportunities for people from every academic and professional background. Your role could involve working to tackle the causes of ill health by improving access to clean water and sanitation facilities. You could help prevent infectious diseases through immunisation programmes, through the use of health technologies such as malaria bed nets, or by encouraging healthy sexual behaviours such as the use of condoms. You could improve the diagnosis of diseases or access to treatment. At an even broader level, global health practitioners develop and improve countries' health systems and train healthcare workers. Work in all of these fields takes many forms, from research at a laboratory or field level, to programmatic technical and implementation work, to administrative and managerial positions. This may sound fantastically exciting – often the work is varied, and requires multi-professional teams of scientists, economists, engineers, doctors and people with local expertise. It is, however, important to be realistic. Whatever job you pursue in global health, much of your day-to-day activity will be the same as any other job, and will involve sitting in an office, writing reports, replying to emails and managing budgets.

Settings

People starting a career in global health need to think about how the world will look in twenty years. The sources of funding, the organisations in which they will work and the nature of the work are all going through a state of change.

Traditionally, global public health has focused on delivering health for the rural poor, often for people who are subsistence farmers. The combined forces of globalisation, urbanisation and economic growth are changing the profile of poverty: the majority of the world's poor people now live in middle income countries (Sumner, 2010). In Kenya, 7 out of 100 children die before their fifth birthday (WHO, 2013), but almost 50 per cent of the population have access to a mobile phone (Aker and Mbiti, 2010). As a result, the nature of global health work is changing, and will increasingly focus on improving the health of the urban poor in middle income countries (WHO, 2010).

Funding for global health is also changing. In 1990, the vast majority of global health funding was delivered in the form of official development assistance – as grants and loans from developed countries to developing countries (Ravishankar *et al.*, 2009). This meant that the traditional setting for global health practitioners was in bilateral donor institutions (such as the UK's Department for International Development), in multilateral organisations (such as the World Health Organization, or the United Nations), or in non-governmental organisations (such as Médecins Sans Frontières or Oxfam[1]). Over the last twenty years, overall funding for global health has almost quadrupled, with a rise in private philanthropy, and new organisations such as the Bill and Melinda Gates Foundation (Ravishankar *et al.*, 2009). As economic growth continues, global health will increasingly be funded through tax incomes (in the same way that public health is funded in the UK and most of Western Europe) and from remittances sent home by wealthy diaspora. We are already seeing this change – the UK government is ending aid to India in recognition of that country's increasing economic and political clout. Despite this, India is home to over one-third of the world's poor people (Agrawal, 2013). The private sector will fill the gap; people starting careers in global health will increasingly have to work in a shifting landscape of social enterprise, private sector and tax-based funding.

Health challenges

The health problems that we tackle also reflect a changing world. Climate change is already affecting global health, and the effects of climate change on health will only get worse (Costello *et al.*, 2009). As countries become more affluent, diets and behaviours are becoming more 'Westernised', often with poor health impacts. To take an example, we know that smoking kills and that around half of all regular cigarette smokers will be killed due to their tobacco use (Doll *et al.*, 2004). One of the key achievements of public health in the Western world in the last twenty-five years has been the gradual reduction in the number of adults who smoke. This is not yet true in the developing world – the number of tobacco smokers has risen drastically in India, China and Africa, and continues to rise. This is creating a time bomb of cancer, heart disease and lung disease. If current patterns continue, smoking will kill around one billion people worldwide in the next hundred years (Peto and Lopez, 2004). Tackling problems like these, through a combination of research, policy and private enterprise, will be a key issue for global public health during our careers.

Achievements

In the last 50 years, life expectancy worldwide has increased from 46.5 years, to 65.2 years (Jong-wook, 2003), an extra 19 years of life for every person born today. That is a remarkable achievement driven by a range of factors, including economic growth and public health progress in water and sanitation, nutrition and vaccination.

Most major achievements in public health are not down to one person, but are the work of decades of concerted effort by thousands of people. As a result, its heroes tend to be underappreciated. Take the eradication of smallpox – a massive global public health effort that ended a disease that has killed millions of people throughout history. This would not have been possible without the laboratory scientists who developed the vaccines, the companies who manufactured it, the organisations that developed supply chains for smallpox vaccines, the politicians and academics who pushed for the international use of smallpox vaccination, and the people on the ground who actually administered the vaccine. The same process has been replicated with polio, and after a twenty-five year effort, we are on the verge of the worldwide eradication of a second human disease.

Despite this, a number of challenges exist. Our global health careers will be driven by climate change, by non-communicable diseases as globalisation and economic growth affect lifestyles, and by inequalities in health outcomes within countries (Frenk and Moon, 2013).

Applicants, skills and qualifications and getting started

Global health is a very competitive world. For almost all positions, a relevant under-graduate degree is essential, as is a variety of volunteering and internship experience. Relevant degrees can take many forms and the skills required in global health are broad. A background in clinical medicine or nursing can be helpful in some circumstances, but a number of other disciplines are equally valuable, including anthropology, statistics, engineering, law, international relations, economics and management, among others.

Increasingly, global health organisations value private-sector experience, so work experience in other fields can be an advantage – you can bring useful professional skills from the worlds of publicity, accounting, media and many others to your global health organisation.

Global public health is not easy, and you need to be prepared to work in settings where the electricity is unreliable, you may not have clean water and you cannot just pop to a supermarket once a week. You may be a long way from your friends and family; you will almost certainly earn less than your contemporaries. At a junior level, you may spend a lot of time jumping between short-term contracts, looking for job security.

In order to work overseas, most organisations want to know that you understand the challenges you will face, that you are able to work effectively in resource-limited settings and in different cultural contexts. For many people, this means that a stint of unpaid volunteering or internship is essential. Be careful of short-term 'voluntourism' programmes, which involve activities such as building schools. These can be exploitative for you (by taking your money for unnecessary work) and exploitative for the host communities (by taking jobs away from host people with more skills and experience). It is far better to get valuable experience with UK-based organisations and develop a set of contacts to identify useful international opportunities.

In order to get started, you should try to develop an understanding of the world of public health – through university courses, public talks and reading around the topic. There is a large online community of academics and professionals working in global public health, and you can use this to find useful articles to read, keep abreast of current events and identify volunteering and internship opportunities. At a university level, student organisations like Medsin and Engineers Without Borders arrange talks, training and summer internships. Getting involved with the leadership team of these organisations can provide you with useful management experience and help you develop your curriculum vitae (CV). At a professional level, organisations like Alma Mata in London and the Royal Society for Public Health allow you to network and meet like-minded individuals. As you read more, find out more about the field and gain more experience, you will undoubtedly find a niche that fits your skills, experience and interests.

Manuelle Hurwitz: working in international development and health for the International Planned Parenthood Federation (IPPF)

IPPF function

The IPPF is a global service provider and a leading advocate of sexual and reproductive health and rights for all. The IPPF was born in the early 1950s thanks to the action of a group of women and men committed to recognising women's right to control their fertility and to increasing access to family planning services. Today, the IPPF is a Federation of 152 Member Associations, working in 172 countries and running 65,000 service points worldwide. Over the years, in line with the International Conference on Population and Development (ICPD) in 1994, the IPPF has broadened its mandate. While contraception remains at the core of IPPF action, its overall aim is to improve the quality of life of individuals by providing and campaigning for sexual and reproductive health and rights through advocacy and services, especially for poor and vulnerable people. The IPPF works to ensure that women are not put at unnecessary risk of injury, illness and death as a result of pregnancy and childbirth, and it supports a woman's right to choose to terminate her pregnancy legally and safely. The IPPF strives to eliminate sexually transmitted infections and to reduce the spread and impact of HIV and AIDS.[2]

The IPPF focuses on reducing gender inequality and reaching vulnerable people who, because of their age, socioeconomic status, sexual orientation, HIV status and other factors, see their human and reproductive rights violated and face barriers in accessing sexual and reproductive health services. As such, the IPPF has identified youth, HIV/AIDS, safe abortion and access to contraceptive and other reproductive health services within a gender- and rights-based approach as its key priorities. In all these areas, IPPF combines a strong advocacy programme with service delivery.

The basis of the IPPF's advocacy is the recognition of sexual and reproductive rights as basic human rights.[3] It is this position that the IPPF, as an NGO, promotes when others too close to national governments may find difficult to explicitly endorse. It is also this stance that informs all areas of IPPF work. As such, one of the IPPF's central commitments is to promote and to provide contraceptive services for all.

The number of women in developing countries who want to delay, space or avoid becoming pregnant, yet are not using effective methods of contraception was estimated at 222 million in 2012.[4] Universal access to, and informed use of effective contraception is the cornerstone to good sexual and reproductive health and to the realisation of people's reproductive rights.[5] Similarly, IPPF Member Associations work in innovative ways to reach out to vulnerable groups, in particular young people, from diverse backgrounds who would otherwise not receive information and services. These services include comprehensive sexuality education; contraception; safe abortion services; sexually transmitted infection (including HIV) prevention, testing and counselling services; prenatal and post-partum services; counselling in sexual abuse, relationships and sexuality.

IPPF's HIV/AIDS programme is equally strong and links prevention with treatment, care and support within an integrated package of sexual and reproductive health services. It also works to reduce HIV-related stigma and discrimination. In both its HIV/AIDS and youth programmes, the IPPF ensures that the voices of young people and people living with HIV/AIDS are included in the decision-making processes that affect their lives.

Another illustration of the IPPF's commitment to sexual and reproductive rights is its commitment to upholding a woman's right to decide the outcome of her pregnancy and to eliminating unsafe abortion, which is a key contributor to maternal mortality worldwide, especially in developing countries. The latest WHO data[6] estimate the number of deaths from unsafe abortions to 47,000 per year in 2008. It is estimated that 21.6 million unsafe abortions took place in 2008, 98 per cent of which were in developing countries.

The IPPF works through six regional offices located in Brussels, Nairobi, Tunis, New York, Kuala Lumpur and New Delhi. The regional offices play a key role providing direct programmatic and financial technical support and monitoring to local IPPF Member Associations, regional advocacy for sexual and reproductive rights, and regional resource mobilisation. Volunteerism is central to the IPPF's ethos and millions of volunteers work with the federation around the world, both in terms of governance and in programme implementation and service delivery.

My route

My path to public health, and specifically sexual and reproductive health and international development, was not unusual in the sense that it combined both passion and sheer luck. From my time in secondary school, I had a special interest in history and human geography, and developed a real thirst for learning about different cultures. This naturally led me to study sociology and social anthropology at Brussels University, where I focused my attention on how culture and values impact on every aspect of people's lives, including socioeconomic order, family relationships / hierarchy, sexuality and health. While my degree in social anthropology gave me sound qualitative research skills, I felt the need to complete my education with stronger quantitative competencies and, thanks to a grant from the British Council, came to England to study medical demography at the London School of Hygiene & Tropical Medicine. I would have never thought this personal interest would lead me to work for a non-governmental organisation (NGO) like the International Planned Parenthood Federation (IPPF).

It would be fair to say that I came to IPPF through chance, although my determination to find a career that would allow me to apply my knowledge and interest in social sciences definitely helped. Following an advertisement in a national newspaper, I successfully applied for a job in the IPPF South Asia Regional Office in 1992. As part of my career progression, I joined the Central Office in 2001 where I worked in different capacities to finally become the Senior Adviser in charge of the abortion programme. I fell into this post both through my personal interest for an issue I saw as too often overlooked due to high political and religious sensitivities, and the opportunity given to me at that time to lead a large programme focusing on reducing unsafe abortion and improving access to safe legal abortion in countries of Eastern Europe, Africa and South and South East Asia.

My role

My current responsibilities are to provide strategic and technical leadership, including the expansion of quality contraceptive and safe abortion services integrated in a broad package of sexual and reproductive health services in IPPF Member Associations' facilities. My work is soundly based on IPPF policy, which states that women and couples have the right to decide the number and spacing of their children, including the right to access contraceptive services and, when an unintended pregnancy has occurred, to have access to safe abortion services.

My specific tasks include ensuring support for IPPF regional offices and country Member Associations in the development of accurate and culturally sensitive messaging; facilitating workshops to explore values surrounding abortion; representing IPPF at external and global meetings and conferences; disseminating the latest technical updates on abortion; monitoring clinics for adherence to WHO and IPPF quality of care standards; and developing and managing programmes and grants. Ensuring access to reliable and affordable contraception to prevent unwanted pregnancy is also a key part of this role, as part of IPPF core mandate. As part of my job, I travel frequently to support Member Associations and monitor clinics. My knowledge of French has allowed me to focus my attention on francophone Africa where the unmet needs are particularly high.

My role is challenging and demands great commitment to the issue, diplomacy and sensitivity to different legal and cultural contexts. The skills required to perform my role are similar to many jobs in the IPPF. These include knowledge in public health, preferably sexual and reproductive health, experience in working in developing countries, strong written and verbal communication skills, programme management, including financial and budgeting skills, resource mobilisation, the ability to work in a team and, of course, a sensitivity to different cultures. While technical knowledge in public and population health is often seen as a major requirement for such role, the need for strong programme and grant management skills cannot be overlooked. A large part of my job consists of developing proposals and bids, overseeing programme implementation and writing reports in line with donors' priorities and requirements.

Challenges

While this is undoubtedly a rewarding job, it comes with many responsibilities and challenges. Like in all large organisations, especially working in the Central Office, it is sometimes difficult to directly see the impact of our work on people's lives. Also, the need to accommodate many different legal and cultural contexts may often require compromises and negotiations, thus the need for flexibility and appreciation of how decisions taken at central and even regional levels can affect the position and sustainability of our local Member Associations in their respective countries. Many of our Member Associations work in fragile, low-resource and restrictive environments, which impact on their capacity to deliver the IPPF programme to the full extent ideally expected from them. This is why regular contacts with the regional offices and travels to Member Associations are needed to better understand and empathise with their situation. On a personal level, the frequency of travels can take its toll on social and family relationships, and it can be very difficult to manage a good work–life balance, especially when you have children. Thankfully, this is now increasingly less of an issue with the opportunities offered by technology to work from home when needed. Last but not least, NGOs like IPPF are vulnerable to changes in the global political scene and in the funding priorities of donors, especially bilateral donors. The need to keep abreast of our external environment and quickly adapt to possible changes while remaining true to our mission and values can be demanding, yet is essential to sustain our action.

Rewards

Yet, in spite of these challenges, the rewards are many and can be truly life enhancing. Positive changes brought from our action and programmes, although sometimes slow and hard to obtain, do happen whether in terms of increasing the capacity of local Member Associations to achieve their objectives, supporting clinics to deliver services to those who need it the most or improving the commitment of the public, policy-makers and media to sexual and reproductive rights. The ultimate reward is to witness or hear from a client, even only once, who has just received a service (HIV/AIDS, family planning, safe abortion, gender-based violence or other) in one of our clinics, or to observe positive changes in global or national laws and policies recognising people's reproductive rights. It is then that statistics and performance data become human and meaningful.

Getting started

Students and professionals looking for a career in public health and specifically in international development in an NGO like the IPPF do not all need to follow a similar path. They may be doctors, nurses, lawyers, social scientists, or others. Of course, most technical and/or managerial posts in international development today require a postgraduate degree either in public health or social sciences such as demography, population and development, or gender studies. Candidates will also need sound technical knowledge in their respective field of interest and strong interpersonal skills. An appreciation of and experience working in developing countries would certainly be a strong asset, as would the knowledge of languages other than English, especially French or Spanish. This can be obtained through professional but also voluntary work or research placement/internships abroad, which have the added advantage of showing one's ability to take initiatives and adaptability. The road to such a career may be long and will therefore require patience, tenacity and good networking skills. It is important to ask for possible internships, send CVs around and contact staff working in fields of particular interest.

The impact of a career like mine may feel like a drop in the ocean and a never-ending task. Yet, it is amazingly rewarding and offers countless opportunities not only in terms of career development but personal fulfilment. Just remember, no one in this job is a hero; all it takes is to be a fellow human being determined to work tirelessly for what he or she believes in.

Notes

1 MSF and Oxfam are large, well-known international NGOs. There are also a huge number of local in-country NGOs that do very important work.
2 IPPF website: www.ippf.org. Accessed 21 February 2013.
3 IPPF. Sexual rights: an IPPF declaration, 2008. Available at: www.ippf.org/resources/publications/sexual-rights-ippf-declaration.
4 Guttmacher Institute. Adding it up: costs and benefits of contraceptive services – estimates for 2012. Available at: www.guttmacher.org/pubs/AIU-2012-estimates.pdf.
5 IPPF website: www.ippf.org. Accessed 21 February 2013.
6 World Health Organization. Unsafe abortion: global and regional estimates of the incidence of unsafe abortion and associated mortality in 2008, 6th edn. World Health Organization. Geneva, Switzerland. 2011. Available at: http://whqlibdoc.who.int/publications/2011/9789241501118_eng.pdf.

References

Agrawal, N. Should rich countries stop sending development aid to India? No. *British Medical Journal*, 346, 73–73. 2013.

Aker, J. and Mbiti, I. *Mobile phones and economic development in Africa*. Center for Global Development, Working Paper 211. 2010.

Costello, A., Abbas, M., Allen, A., Ball, S., Bell, S., Bellamy, R., Friel, S., Groce, N., Johnson, A., Kett, M., Lee, M., Levy, C., Maslin, M., McCoy, D., McGuire, B., Montgomery, H., Napier, D., Pagel, C., Patel, J., de Oliveira, J.A.P., Redclift, N., Rees, H., Rogger, D., Scott, J., Stephenson, J., Twigg, J., Wolff, J. and Patterson, C. Managing the health effects of climate change. *The Lancet*, 373, 1693–1733. 2009.

Doll, R., Peto, R., Boreham, J. and Sutherland, I. Mortality in relation to smoking: 50 years' observations on male British doctors. *British Medical Journal*, 328, 1519. 2004.

Frenk, J. and Moon, S. Governance challenges in global health. *The New England Journal of Medicine*, 368, 936–942. 2013.

Jong-wook, L. Global health improvement and WHO: shaping the future. *The Lancet*, 362, 2083–2088. 2003.

Peto, R. and Lopez, A. The future worldwide health effects of current smoking patterns. *Tobacco and Public Health: Science and Policy*, 281–286. 2004.

Ravishankar, N., Gubbins, P., Cooley, R.J., Leach-Kemon, K., Michaud, C.M., Jamison, D.T. and Murray, C.J. Financing of global health: tracking development assistance for health from 1990 to 2007. *The Lancet*, 373, 2113–2124. 2009.

Sumner, A. *Global poverty and the new bottom billion: what if three-quarters of the world's poor live in middle-income countries?* Institute of Development Studies, Working Paper 349, 01–43. 2010.

World Health Organization (WHO) *Why urban health matters*. Geneva, WHO: 2010.

World Health Organization (WHO) *World health statistics: mortality and global health estimates*. Available online at: http://apps.who.int/gho/data/node.main.2?lang=en. Accessed 30 April 2013.

11 UK voluntary and community sector organisations

Paul Lincoln; Claire Everett and Susan Lloyd

Introduction to this setting

Voluntary and community sector (VCS) organisations and charities have been working to improve the health of the population for many centuries. Increasingly, they are being used to deliver direct care as well as supplement the work of health services and local government. They often play a major role in advocacy for the cause that they represent and sometimes work in partnership with other like-minded organisations to lobby politicians in support of their shared priorities.

EXAMPLES OF PUBLIC HEALTH PRACTITIONER ROLES IN THIS SETTING

The contributions here offer a taster of the major role this often unrecognised sector plays in efforts to improve the health and wellbeing of the population in the UK as well as its international influence. You will witness some of the substantial opportunities the sector offers to people who want to work to see change for the better in the public's health.

Paul Lincoln, Chief Executive, UK Health Forum

According to the Association of Chief Executives of the Voluntary Sector (ACEVO), the UK charity sector consists of over 900,000 organisations with a combined turnover of £157 billion, a workforce of over 1.6 million and combined assets of £244 billion and the capacity to mobilise a quarter of the population to volunteer formally at least once a month. The VCS is, in effect, 'organised civil society' or organised community action – a hugely significant economic and social force.

Charities are often described as non-governmental organisations (NGOs) and are not-for-profit organisations that are registered and regulated by the Charity Commission. The sector is also often referred to as part of the third sector and civil society.

In the UK, the VCS is developed around serving people's needs and often fills the gaps not identified or provided for in the public sector. The sector is very diverse with charities of all sizes working at local, national and international levels. They tackle a wide range of needs and issues on health, social, economic and environmental concerns.

The sector is very diverse. It consists of charities that are research organisations, campaigning organisations or provide services for people – and often a mixture of these roles. In the health sector Cancer Research UK (CRUK) and the British Heart Foundation (BHF) fund significant amounts of research, mainly clinical, and are fundamentally patient-interest organisations. However, they are becoming increasingly engaged in public health matters. Other charities such as Action on Smoking and Health (ASH) campaign to reduce smoking and tackle the excesses of the tobacco industry. The National Children's Bureau and Age UK represent the needs of children, young people and older people, respectively. Many groups deal directly with equity issues such as the Men's Health Forum or the Race Equality Foundation. Others tackle the social, economic or environmental causes of ill health such as the child poverty action group; or Sustain (alliance for better food and farming) and the Soil Association, which work to create healthier food supply from the farm to the plate; or Friends of the Earth (FoE), which tackles sustainable development and climate change – arguably the world's biggest public health challenge. Many of these organisations are in the business of public health, but would not necessarily perceive themselves as being so.

Charities also vary enormously in size; increasingly, the sector is made up of fewer bigger national charities that are dominated by particular organisations with strong public brands. The sector also works at all levels – local, national and international. International development is a key public health area and the Millennium Development Goals have enabled a focus on major public health issues, which require action that necessitates building a competent, active non-governmental civil society.

Charities are often started in response to a pressing social problem that is not being addressed, sufficiently prioritised or not in the right way. Action on Smoking and Health (ASH) was started as a consequence of the Royal College of Physicians' (RCP) report on tobacco, which identified the links between tobacco and smoking, and the need for an independent charity to tackle the vested interests of the tobacco industry, which, at the time, was free to market its products without any restrictions.

The sector is mainly funded by public donations, legacies and fund-raising events. The sector's mandate emerges from representing under-represented communities and interests that are not addressed. Charities have to pass a public benefit test and are legally required by the Charity Commission to produce an annual public benefit statement of their value to society.

Contribution to improving health and reducing health inequalities

ACEVO published a report in 2010 entitled 'The Organised Efforts of Society' which summarises three key roles for the sector in relation to public health:

- leadership, voice and advocacy;
- informing and shaping policy and strategy;
- designing, delivering and supporting services.

These multifaceted roles of the VCS in public health are manifest in many ways. VCS organisations are close to population groups most in need and those less well reached or served by public services. They often campaign and champion the needs and concerns of these groups, particularly the vulnerable and dispossessed seeking equality, tackling health inequalities, and seeking social and environmental justice. Charities promote the case for social change. They often tackle the wider social determinants of health and are interested in promoting wellbeing. Some NGOs directly challenge the vested interests of the tobacco, alcohol and processed food industries, which damage the public's health.

VCS organisations often set the social policy agenda and are very active politically. However, under charity law they have to be apolitical and thus seek to inform and gain support from all political parties for change. Increasingly, they work together in alliances such as the smoke-free tobacco control alliance or the alcohol and health alliance. There are also many umbrella organisations that seek to broker common advocacy positions and the power of collective action. These charities include the UK Health Forum (previously the National Heart Forum), which promotes the primary prevention of all linked avoidable chronic conditions and Sustain, the food, agricultural and health alliance.

VCS organisations often take on scrutiny/challenge roles of public-sector organisations, through organisations that represent patients and key groups often providing a reality check for public services. Recent developments include Health Watch, which will scrutinise local public services and have a place on local Health and Wellbeing Boards. Other charities such as ASH, the Alcohol Health Alliance, Sustain and UK Health Forum closely monitor and challenge the health-damaging actions of the alcohol, tobacco, processed food and marketing industries. These organisations are a countervailing force to industries that potentially damage health at a population level. This is necessary because government is often compromised and conflicted by other factors such as economic interests. This is an area of work that the VCS can undertake in ways that no other part of the publicly funded public health system can. An example would be the Campaign on Action on Salt and Health (CASH), which challenges industry and government to reduce salt in processed foods.

VCS organisations are often expert organisations and have specialist expertise on disease and social conditions in addition to providing key insights into population groups. They also have independent information services and dedicated networks of interested parties and the key activists. Many provide resources to patients and sufferers and carers on all health issues.

Many of the larger charities such as CRUK and BHF commission large amounts of research on treatments and increasingly on prevention. Often this is in collaboration with the main government-funded research organisations such as the Medical Research Council and the Wellcome Foundation.

Many charities are providers of services through their own funding or through funding from the public purse. Many charities are able to provide these services through volunteers. In recent years social enterprises have been rapidly developing and new forms of not-for-profit third-sector organisations are possible. The government has encouraged these developments as part of its vision for the 'Big Society' whereby public services are transferred from the state and provided by these new types of organisations and charities. The advantage of this idea is that they are closer to key groups and have lower transactional costs for the public purse, and hence are cheaper and more cost-effective providers.

Charities are highly credible and trusted messengers. They are values driven and immersed in equality and in equity, an issue that is in the DNA of the workers in the sector. The goals are social, human and environmental justice. They are in the business of social results and are highly focused on achieving social outcomes. They are thus dedicated, flexible, innovative and entrepreneurial, and have access to the neediest groups in society.

Opportunities for careers

Despite the well-recognised contribution of the sector to improving population health, regrettably there is currently no career framework for public health in this sector. There has been no strategic consideration about the developments of careers in this sector despite its considerable value to the public health movement and its considerable achievements in improving public health.

However, recently there have been a number of potentially promising developments. Public Health England (2013) in its first document on the public health workforce, for which it now has as a prime responsibility, pointed out the need for strategic workforce development in the sector. The VCS is seen as part of the wider public health workforce.

Further, with the reforms to the health and social care sector in England the new NHS strategy Transforming the Workforce (2012) offers some possibilities. The needs of the sector may begin to be partly addressed by the new agency, Health Education England, which will oversee all basic and post-basic training and education of the health workforce, and integrate this with social care and public health, and the work of the local authority and the third sector. Much will depend upon the new local education and training boards (local Health Education organisations). Ideally, they should have links with the VCS and be supporting such developments, especially between the statutory and voluntary sectors.

Some public health achievements by the sector

The following organisations are powerful alliances that unite the charity world, and their collective power is harnessed and forms powerful social movements.

- The HIV/AIDS groups such as the Terrence Higgins Trust have been very effective in preventing the spread of HIV infections among the general population, and gay and bisexual groups. These groups have been very effective advocates for developing public services and are influential messengers for key population groups.
- The Campaign for Action on Salt and Health, in collaboration with other NGOs such as WHICH? and the UK Health Forum, has ensured that the government sets a national salt reduction target and successfully put pressure on industry to reformulate processed foods to reduce salt.
- The Stroke Association effectively campaigned for the government to fund a marketing campaign to increase public awareness of the early signs of a stroke and encouraged the government to produce a national stroke strategy. Prior to this, stroke prevention and early intervention had been a long-standing neglected area. Many of the chronic disease organisations have provided expert advice and organised advocacy campaigns for cardiovascular disease, dementia, cancers, diabetes and obesity.
- ASH was formed after the Royal College of Physicians produced their seminal report 'Smoking and Health' and has successfully campaigned for the progressive regulation of the tobacco industry and nicotine products. Most recently, it has helped secure restrictions on marketing and to prevent smoking in enclosed public spaces and is currently campaigning to introduce standardised packaging for all tobacco products.
- Sustrans (sustainable transport) is an expert charity that has advised national and local government on promoting cycling as a right and strongly advocated the links with health. A national cycling network has been established and increased funding for cycle ways.
- The Child Poverty Action Group has relentlessly campaigned for the eradication of child poverty and ensured that it is a primary public policy goal. It has also supported policies such as the minimum wage.
- Umbrella groups such as the UK Health Forum work in alliance with other charities, professional and academic groups to campaign for action on restricting the marketing of foods high in fat, salt and sugar until after the 9pm watershed, and for the universal front-of-pack, nutritional, easy-to-read traffic light labelling.
- The Alcohol Health Alliance has put the case for minimum unit pricing of alcohol on the political agenda and will continue to make the case until it is introduced.

What it is like working in the sector?

The sector is strongly driven by public interest values, justice and fairness. This is the primary motivation of those who work in the sector. There is a sense that anything is possible and the flexibility of the sector enables imaginative and radical thinking in ways that are often constrained in the public and private sectors. The bottom line is social change and much progressive thinking is born in the sector. Social reform and innovation are key characteristics.

Many small VCS organisations are highly focused on achieving social policy goals, and thus are very creative and innovative. They are not as constrained as the public sector and are thus able to use novel approaches to finding solutions. They are not as restricted as the public sector in terms of the political environment in which they work, and have more freedom to operate and articulate causes although they must be apolitical in their work. Their mandate comes from their members and the communities they serve.

The UK coalition government is keen to promote a diversity of providers for public services and encourage social enterprises. The VCS are seen as agents of social change and part of the Big Society[1] vision whereby more power is given to communities and community organisations. Many new organisational structures are now being set up for these new organisations to encourage social entrepreneurs. Charities and not-for-profit, non-state organisations are being seen as a means to deliver and transform public services. Much greater emphasis is now being placed on the type of social value in ways that charities measure success.

How to start?

There is no standard route and no career framework in the VCS as yet. However, there is plenty of scope if you are interested. If you are already in a public health career, then consider spending some time in a charity either through employment or via a secondment or work attachment.

Generally, working for a charity will present opportunities, in particular campaigns, policy development, and advocacy and research. The Third Sector advertises jobs weekly on its website and in its magazine.

Volunteers are always welcomed and it can lead to work opportunities. Look for progressive charities, and think about the wider determinants of health and health inequalities and the charity's mission.

You can also approach the local education and training boards (LETB), which should have websites giving details of training opportunities.

Claire Everett, Regional Commissioning Manager, Food for Life Partnership and Sue Lloyd, Specialist in Public Health and Nutrition

The Food for Life Partnership (FFLP) is a third sector organisation, providing a health improvement programme that uses schools as a setting to encourage and enable positive eating behaviours. Our key objective is to empower schools and their communities to develop the opportunities, confidence and abilities required for children and families to access healthy and sustainable food, and to provide the skills and knowledge that enable them to make informed food choices and lead healthy lives.

From 2007 to 2012, the FFLP was fully funded by the Big Lottery Fund to develop and implement a national programme aimed at transforming school food culture. The programme is delivered through an awards framework that takes a place-based approach to supporting schools and their caterers in improving food leadership and school food culture, food quality, food education, and community and partnership links. Success of the programme during this initial period has led to further support from the Big Lottery Fund being confirmed until 2015 to fund our core team and enable expansion of the programme into new settings, such as early years, care homes and workplaces. The schools-based element of the programme is continuing, now funded in local areas via public health commissioning.

By using the school as a community hub and setting for early intervention, the FFLP framework helps children to form healthy eating habits, and provides them and their parents with access to practical learning and food skills, giving them greater control over their current and future diets. The programme covers many aspects of food, including developing pupil voice in the planning and delivery of a whole-school food policy; increasing teacher confidence in teaching food growing and cooking skills to children; enabling schools to make the most of farm visits to connect with where food comes from; and working with caterers to ensure that food served in schools is responsibly sourced, healthy and appetising. In this way, the programme outcomes contribute towards improving healthy life expectancy, including what happens at the start of life and how well people live across the life course.

Independent evaluation studies carried out during the initial five-year phase of the FFLP demonstrated positive impacts across health improvement and the wider determinants of health. As a result of engagement in the programme, a 28 per cent increase was seen in the proportion of primary school-age children reporting eating five portions of fruit and vegetables per day, and 45 per cent of parents reported eating more fruit and vegetables as a result of the programme (Orme et al., 2011). The evaluators reported that there were 'statistically significant associations between healthy eating and FFLP-related behaviours such as participation in cooking and growing at school or at home; participation in farm and sustainable food learning; and attitudes to school food' (Orme et al., 2011). Importantly, schools engaged in the FFLP integrate food skills and education into curriculum time, so that all children are able to benefit instead of only the proportion that opts to take part in extra-curricular clubs and activities.

One method of tackling health inequalities nationally is through the provision of free school meals for children from disadvantaged families. However, 20 per cent of eligible primary school children and 30 per cent of eligible secondary school children (Nelson et al., 2010) do not take up this entitlement for varying reasons, including stigma and the lure of unhealthier food options. Free school meal take-up increased by an average of 13 percentage points in FFLP primary schools and by 20 percentage points in secondary schools (Orme et al., 2011). Collectively, the evaluation studies have shown how the FFLP supports all six recommendations from the 2010 Marmot Review 'Fair Society, Healthy Lives' (Marmot, 2010) and, as a programme accessible to all schools, its effectiveness has been particularly evident in schools within areas of high social deprivation (Orme et al., 2011), demonstrating proportionate universalism and helping to 'close the gap' for disadvantaged children in terms of their health and academic attainment (Teeman *et al.*, 2011).

The FFLP's four original partners – the Soil Association, Garden Organic, Focus on Food and the Health Education Trust – were joined in 2013 by a fifth partner, the Royal Society for Public Health. The programme is led by the Soil Association, coordinated by a central office-based team, which provides overall management, policy direction, communications and administration of the awards programme. Regional home-based commissioning managers develop programmes with local authority public health teams, and local programme managers coordinate implementation of these. The partner organisations contribute to on-going development of the FFLP and lead training for school staff within locally commissioned programmes.

Across the FFLP team, at national level we are working with, and continually building relationships with, the Department for Education, Department of Health and Public Health England, fellow third-sector organisations and occasionally private-sector organisations. At regional and local levels we develop our programmes with public health and other local authority teams, work closely with schools and may form links with local NHS colleagues such as community dieticians. At community level, our schools form hubs of good food culture reaching out to local voluntary organisations, and, importantly, parents and families.

As one of four regional commissioning managers, Claire's role is to develop programmes with local authority public health commissioners, which they then contract the FFLP to implement and manage. Although the FFLP developed as a schools-focused, education- and skills-based intervention, the practical outcomes that the programme achieves in public health terms are very clear. It is the success of this work that has created opportunities for the FFLP to expand into new settings under the Soil Association's 'Good food for all' strategy. Our transition from a Lottery-funded to a locally commissionable programme coincided with the transition of public health from the NHS into local authorities and the formation of Health and Wellbeing Boards, which is creating closer working between local authority teams, as well as with community and voluntary organisations. The FFLP programme provides a great practical example of how council officers from many disciplines beyond public health and education – including catering services, allotments teams and leisure providers – can integrate their work to improve population health and wellbeing. The transition of public health into local authorities has brought with it new accountability structures for public health teams, along with budgetary changes and new procurement processes – all of which we have to be very familiar with when developing programmes.

During the development of local programmes, as commissioning managers, we form close strategic relationships with the public health team, working together to tackle the needs identified in the Joint Strategic Needs Assessments and the targets presented in the Health and Wellbeing Strategies. This results in each commissioned programme being built around local need, increasing its effectiveness and impact within that locality. Throughout programmes, we work in partnership with our public health commissioners to continue to develop our evidence base, ensuring appropriate monitoring and evaluation according to programme capacity and local priorities.

When a programme is commissioned, a local programme manager is recruited to manage and coordinate delivery. After being interviewed, usually jointly by the commissioning manager and local public health officer, the local programme manager is line-managed by the commissioning manager, thus becoming part of the FFLP team. By being part of a national network of local programme managers, learning and experience from all programmes can be combined with local knowledge and applied effectively to the local setting. Although hands-on programme management is a big part of this role, the local programme manager remit also extends beyond this to strategic influencing and development. Being able to convey and demonstrate the successes and challenges of changing food culture in a meaningful way to multiple stakeholders – whether children, parents, school cooks, head teachers or directors of public health – requires insightful understanding of what each hopes to achieve from the programme. A local programme manager needs a good understanding of school structures and functioning, public health issues, data collection and evaluation, and other local services or organisations that may be partnered with or signposted to. Furnished with this knowledge, opportunities for collaboration can be developed and, by working in partnership to build on existing structures and projects, innovative ways are often found to add value and increase impact.

Members of the FFLP team come from a wide variety of backgrounds with diverse areas of expertise, including nutrition, environmental sciences, sustainable development, teaching, farming, zoology and animal welfare. The great thing about the FFLP programme is that each of these areas is valued within it and so, by learning from each other, we are continually strengthening our approach and work. Of course, our common ground is that we all share a strong passion for good food and a belief that everyone is entitled to the education, knowledge and practical skills that enable them to experience this for themselves. A key emerging theme in public health that is continually gathering pace and recognition is the relationship between health and sustainable development or ecology. The FFLP embodies this thinking whether through highlighting the simultaneous environmental and health benefits of eating less meat and more local, seasonal, organically grown vegetables, or through partnering with active transport initiatives that encourage walking or cycling instead of driving to increase physical activity levels at the same time as reducing carbon emissions. One thing that is seen across many third-sector organisations is that employees live to their values. In our case, this means eating responsibly sourced food, living a healthy lifestyle and, for many of us, creating time to grow and cook food as part of our everyday routines.

While not everyone in the FFLP team has formal public health training, we hold a wide range of experience in this area. A good basic understanding of key aspects such as whole-settings approaches to health promotion, behaviour change, epidemiology and how this relates to evidence-based practice and policy development is a useful starting point, and is built upon daily in practice. As well as a vast array of knowledge and experience, the team, and each individual, possesses a multitude of skills. Good communication is vital – for example, within a single day you could be writing and emailing a newsletter to local authority public health colleagues, meeting with a Director of Public Health and presenting at a conference. With this in mind, we need to multitask continually but also to hold strong prioritisation skills and be able to manage our time around focusing on the most pressing issues. Proactivity is another asset, along with the ability to respond to political or economic change as competing influences on public health emerge locally and nationally. Confidence is essential and, as with many careers, is something that develops with time as you immerse yourself in a role, programme or setting.

Working as a team is incredibly important to the success of a programme like the FFLP, but equally necessary is an ability to be able to work and make decisions independently. A large number of our team work remotely, and we strive hard to support each other in finding a balance between valuing time spent working from our home office and our enthusiasm for being out and about meeting internal and external colleagues. We are in constant contact with people by telephone and email, and have regular team catch-ups and opportunities to meet with and develop ideas with all partners.

Achievements of the FFLP team are seen in many ways. In the broadest sense, achievement is evident in the continued funding and commissioning of the programme. One of the challenges often faced by third-sector organisations is short-term funding and the ongoing need to reinvent projects and apply to new funding streams to secure future funds. The FFLP's success in transitioning from charity funding to public health commissioning is therefore a great achievement, and while we continue to seek funding to embed our existing local programmes over longer term periods and explore opportunities to develop new ones, there is a definite sense of this being a positive developmental process.

Our evidence base demonstrates another aspect of achievement through the impact we are having on improving children's health and wellbeing. Through the associated Food for Life Catering Mark scheme, 760,000 meals are now served each day by caterers who have been audited to ensure they are taking positive steps to serve freshly prepared food that is free from undesirable additives and GM ingredients, meet high standards of provenance and traceability, and source food that is better for the environment and animal welfare; they are also taking steps to offer healthier menus. Some 33 per cent of awarded caterers have achieved our silver and gold awards. Among more detailed criteria, these awards ensure that menus are seasonal; a range of local, organic and fair trade produce is sourced; no fish is served from the Marine Conservation Society 'fish to avoid' list; non-meat dishes are promoted; information about where the food has come from is on display; and training is provided for all staff. Catering Mark accredited meals are served across a range of sectors, from public-sector nurseries, schools and hospitals to private-sector sports stadiums, care homes and workplaces.

The FFLP has also received awards in recognition of our work. In 2011, we were proud recipients of the BBC Radio 4 Derek Cooper Award, which recognises 'unsung heroes, whose work has increased our access to, and knowledge and appreciation of, good food'. Continued success of the FFLP as we developed our commissionable models in 2012 led to us being awarded a Health Promotion and Community Wellbeing Award from the Royal Society for Public Health for our work in the field of health and wellbeing.

At all levels within the FFLP team there is a strong desire to make a difference to people's lives. We recognise that we are unable to transform food choices and behaviours overnight, and that people and settings are at very different starting points. However, the small, step-by-step changes we encourage accumulate to make big differences. This is consistently reinforced by seeing progress made by schools in achieving awards, comments made by teachers about the difference the FFLP has made to their pupils and staff, and the look on a child's face as he or she harvests their first red tomato or sees their hand-kneaded loaf of bread rise.

The governance and sheer size of some public-sector institutions can mean change is sometimes slow to emerge, but smaller third-sector organisations (whether national or community) are often able to drive ideas forward much more quickly and it is very rewarding to be a part of this. People working in the not-for-profit sector are always incredibly passionate about what they do, and we often consider ourselves lucky to be paid to do work we enjoy and from which we gain a lot of satisfaction. In relation to this, though, salaries are sometimes lower and, due to funding constraints, contracts may be less secure or short term. However, as you gain experience and move from working on specific projects to a more central role, long-term security can be developed when positions are integrated into an organisation instead of being reliant on a particular funding source. Looked at in a positive sense, this can be a very motivating environment to work in, and one that creates determination and purpose.

Many people enter work in this setting because they like the practical, hands-on elements but, as in many careers, this may have to be left behind as you progress into strategy, planning, research and management-focused roles. The more academic roles will suit some, but others may find it difficult to leave the practical aspects behind. In a good organisation, however, all members of the team will be encouraged to remain in close contact with what is happening 'on the ground' and have opportunities to take time away from their routine job to enjoy and connect with this.

Health improvement work in public health links closely to the social and environmental determinants of health, and to policies and organisations concerned with physical activity, food and community development, which extend beyond public-sector capacity to the third sector. Coupled with the Big Society intentions of the coalition government, which aim to increase public service roles for not-for-profit organisations, it is an exciting time for the third sector in public health.

One of the best things you can do if you are interested in working in this area is to gain experience in a number of different settings. Paid or voluntary work in schools and local authorities, through to a community kitchen or local food-growing project, provides great experience. Also think about your spread of theoretical knowledge combined with practical experience – having different types of knowledge and experience in different areas is often enough to get a foot in the door, and showing a willingness to learn, and ability to learn quickly, is really important. Careers in public health-related third-sector organisations are incredibly challenging and exciting, and, in return for effort, enthusiasm and commitment, highly energising and rewarding.

Note

1   An initiative introduced by the coalition government to promote empowerment of local people and communities.

References

Marmot, M. *Fair Society, Healthy Lives – Strategic Review of Health Inequalities in England post-2010 (The Marmot Review)*. London, University College London. February 2010.

Nelson, M., Nicholas, J., Wood, L., Lever, E., Simpson and Baker, B. *Fifth Annual Survey of Take Up of School Lunches in England*. 2010. Available online at: www.childrensfood trust.org.uk/assets/research-reports/fifth_annual_survey2009–2010_full_report.pdf. Accessed 26 May 2014.

Orme, J., Jones, M., Kimberlee, R., Weitkamp, E., Salmon, D., Dailami, N., Morley, A. and Morgan, J. *Food for Life Partnership Evaluation. University of the West of England and Cardiff University*. 2011. Available online at: http://eprints.uwe.ac.uk/14456/. Accessed 26 May 2014.

Teeman, D., Featherston, G., Sims, D. and Sharp, C. *Qualitative Impact Evaluation of the Food for Life Partnership*. National Foundation for Educational Research. 2011. Available online at: www.nfer.ac.uk/nfer/publications/BINT01/BINT01_home.cfm? publicationID=575&title=Qualitative%20impact%20evaluation%20of%20the%20 Food%20for%20Life%20Partnership%20programme. Accessed 26 May 2014.

Additional reading

Campbell's adaptation of Dahlgren and Whitehead's health map: see Campbell, F. (ed.) *The social determinants of health and the role of local government*. London: IDeA, 2010.

Rayner, G. and Lang, T. *Ecological public health: reshaping the conditions for good health*, Oxford: Routledge, 2012.

Part 4

Getting into public health

Fiona Sim and Jenny Wright

Having read about the settings in which public health specialists and practitioners work and some of the functions they carry out, this part describes ways in which you might start your career in public health. It presents contributors' perspectives on undergraduate and postgraduate courses, being on the public health specialist training scheme and approaches to the development of public health competence. It concludes with a description of what to do next, how to help yourself and how you can make your public health career a reality. The subjects discussed are:

- undergraduate and postgraduate education;
- public health training scheme;
- public health development; and
- how to get going, what to do next.

12 | Undergraduate and postgraduate education

Jane Wills; Helen Hogan

Introduction

The contributors in this chapter cover what it is like to undertake formal Public Health courses at a university at either undergraduate or postgraduate levels, what to expect and what to look for when you apply. For those who would like more information on courses at specific universities, as well as checking out each university's prospectus, visit the UK Public Health Careers website at www.phorcast.org.uk.

WHAT TO EXPECT FROM PUBLIC HEALTH UNDERGRADUATE AND POSTGRADUATE COURSES

Jane Wills, Professor of Public Health

Undergraduate courses

Studying Public Health may be at undergraduate or postgraduate level. At undergraduate level programmes introduce students to key concepts and principles such as those of equity and sustainability. Students will learn about the social determinants of health and develop core skills in measuring health and epidemiology, analysing research evidence and programme planning. Such courses may often be part of a suite of awards that include Health Studies and Health Promotion as these all share aims to improve the health of individuals, communities and populations. Students who study Public Health as their first degree generally have an interest in health but do not want to pursue a vocational degree such as Nursing or another clinical profession. Undergraduate courses in Public Health remain relatively uncommon in UK universities.

Postgraduate courses

At postgraduate level, Public Health may be studied as part of an award leading to a degree of Master of Science (M.Sc.) or a Master of Public Health (MPH).

Academically, there is no difference between the two. An MPH is regarded as a vocational degree, usually, but not always with a curriculum based on the syllabus of the UK Faculty of Public Health, and it is intended to support the first part of training for those who will take up management and leadership roles in public health. Normally, those who study an MPH will hold a relevant professional qualification or have professional or relevant work experience, whether in Medicine or in another field. Although public health practice is now multidisciplinary, its contemporary origins are as a medical specialty and so most of the longer established MPH and M.Sc. courses are at universities that have medical schools. An M.Sc. in Public Health is regarded as an academic degree with a focus on critical analysis of key concepts and theories, research and evidence. Most of these courses will cover the domains of public health identified by the Faculty of Public Health – health improvement, health protection and service improvement – and some courses indicate a particular emphasis on one area. For example, there are numerous courses that are described as M.Sc. Public Health *and* Health Promotion.

In the 1970s the Department of Health invested pump-priming money to set up postgraduate diploma health promotion courses at Leeds Metropolitan University and London South Bank University and later the University of the West of England, and there are now many postgraduate courses that regard themselves as vocational courses in health promotion, and tend to attract applicants who are already working in public health-related roles, such as smoking cessation adviser or physical activity coordinator.

Typically, a Master's course in Public Health will have a wide variety of students with different disciplinary backgrounds that may include science subjects or social science. The majority will have professional experience in the health services as a doctor, nurse or midwife or other clinical professional, but students also come from dietetics, environmental health, pharmacy and health intelligence, and other health and social care professional areas. Increasingly, students come from work in local authorities such as working with children and families or in leisure services. It is this mix of backgrounds that makes Public Health courses so fascinating and as students begin to adopt a new professional identity of public health they also identify opportunities for future collaborative working with and between their original disciplines.

Secondments

Many students will be seconded from their place of work to study part-time, because deeper public health knowledge is seen as a central part of their role or development. Others may be part of a regional training scheme for public health specialists. Students also choose to study Public Health who are considering changing career, their interest often prompted by the personal or professional challenges of encouraging healthier lifestyles. My university course has several students who have been involved with voluntary sector organisations working on particular issues that have included HIV and sexual health, disability issues and literacy. This reflects the history of health promotion, which very much started as a social movement driven by those involved with black and minority health issues, women's health and sexual health.

Students who are seconded by their employer normally return to their role on completing the course, but often take on specialist roles such as, for example, Specialist Midwife for HIV, Health Visitor for Gypsy, Roma and Travellers, Health Protection Specialist or Screening Coordinator. Many students will work in public health departments with specialised roles in relation to a priority area such as obesity or sexual health. Increasingly, graduating students may find new roles in the private health sector or in marketing, including working on health communications and healthy living.

POSTGRADUATE OPPORTUNITIES FOR STUDYING PUBLIC HEALTH

Helen Hogan, Clinical Lecturer

Introduction

Postgraduate courses in Public Health have been an essential element of professional training in Public Health since the early 1900s. The first fully fledged Master's programmes emerged in the 1970s (Fee and Acheson, 1991) and today there are over seventy universities in the UK offering such courses, including Master of Science (M.Sc.) in Public Health, Master of Public Health (MPH) degrees or degrees specialising in an aspect of public health such as population nutrition, health services management or environmental health ('FindAMasters'[1]).

These courses are attracting a wide range of clinical and non-clinical applicants who regard postgraduate training in the relevant knowledge, skills and attitudes, drawing on the latest thinking and research in the field, an excellent preparation for a career in public health. Current courses vary in structure, both in terms of the array of modules on offer and the balance between research, face-to-face teaching and experience in practical settings. An M.Sc. degree tends to be regarded as a qualification that focuses on the theoretical underpinnings of the science of public health, the development of research and evaluative skills, and the ability to undertake a piece of independent research in the form of a dissertation. The MPH encourages the application of theoretical knowledge to contemporary public health problems, planning and managing public health interventions, coupled with practical exposure to the public health working environment. However, in the UK, these courses tend to have overlapping content and there is really little distinction in content or status of the two degrees based on their name alone. The Public Health Online Resource for Careers, Skills and Training (PHORCaST)[2] provides information on postgraduate courses to guide graduates interested in pursuing careers in public health and has produced a report (available on its website) which maps professional public health competencies on to course content for a number of Master's-level degrees.

Course content

A student on an M.Sc. or MPH course should expect to cover the main pillars of public health, including health promotion, environmental health, communicable diseases, health services management, social policy and health economics. Teaching will also be geared to developing proficiency in statistics, epidemiology and the critical appraisal of evidence. Traditional Master's courses attract 180 UK credits and usually take one year full-time or two years part-time to complete. Many courses offer students the prospect of obtaining a postgraduate certificate for 60 credits of learning and a postgraduate diploma for 120 credits. The full 180 credits then are awarded only to those students who also complete a dissertation.

Distance learning

An increasingly popular alternative to the conventional face-to-face Master's is to undertake the degree by distance learning. For some students, the greater flexibility afforded by being able to study within their own time and having up to five years to complete the degree, make this mode of study an attractive option. This is particularly the case at a time when, due to the economic downturn, employers may be reluctant to hold jobs open for a year or let an employee move to half-time in order to undertake further studies. Therefore, a growing number of universities that offer conventional Master's courses in Public Health now also offer distance learning courses.

Getting on to postgraduate courses

Those considering undertaking a postgraduate course in Public Health should initially ask themselves if they have a passion for improving health at a population level, whether they can communicate ideas well in the written form and possess some basic mathematical skills. Most postgraduate courses require that applicants hold at least a Class 2.2 degree in a health-related subject and it is usually seen as an advantage also to have gained some work experience in public health. This experience need not just be within a conventional public health setting but could include voluntary work, internship, working with non-governmental organisations or within the health service as a clinician or manager. If applicants do not have the required academic qualifications, but do have extensive work experience or can demonstrate their ability to cope with a course at this level, then their applications may be assessed on an individual basis to see if a special case might be made for the award of a place on the course. Even if in doubt about your eligibility to apply for a particular course, it may be worthwhile making an enquiry to the admissions office.

What it might lead to

The Master's degree may prepare a graduate either for work within a traditional public health setting or for a future academic career. Those who wish to develop their research skills further are likely to look for opportunities to undertake a Ph.D. As an alternative, the Doctorate in Public Health (Dr.P.H.), a relatively new degree, is designed to create leaders in the field of public health through exposure to research combined with leadership and management training. The intention is that graduates are able both to conduct and critically evaluate research, and are also equipped to take a role in shaping public health policy. Unlike a Ph.D., where a student spends the majority of their time engaged in research, a Dr.P.H. has a larger taught component, a requirement to complete an organisational and policy analysis, as well as under-taking a research project. The degree is normally awarded after three years' full-time enrolment and entry requirements usually include a clinical or professional qualification or a Master's degree, and relevant work experience.

The impact of the expansion of postgraduate provision on the wider public health workforce is unknown, career tracking at both national and university level being poor ('Unistats'[3]). The complexity of this process is made more difficult by the fact that many students have already spent time working in public health before application. Our experience at the London School of Hygiene & Tropical Medicine is that the vast majority of graduates will go on to careers with links to public health in healthcare organisations, local and national government or non-governmental organisations, either within the UK or internationally.

Notes

1 FindAMasters. Available online at: www.findamasters.com/search/courses.aspx?keywords=public+health. Accessed 24 April 2014.
2 Public Health Online Resource for Careers, Skills and Training (PHORCaST). Available online at: www.phorcast.org.uk. Accessed 24 April 2014.
3 Unistats. Available online at: http://unistats.direct.gov.uk. Accessed 24 April 2014.

Reference

Fee, A. and Acheson, R. (eds) *A History of Education in Public Health*. Oxford: Oxford University Press, 1991.

13 Public health specialist training scheme

Amy Potter

Introduction

The UK has a formal training scheme for those public health practitioners who wish to become specialists in public health and proceed to consultant status. Northern Ireland runs its own recruitment. For Scotland, England and Wales there is a single annual recruitment round for suitably qualified individuals, which includes the armed forces. The training scheme is open to applicants from medical and non-medical backgrounds. For further information, visit either the UK Faculty of Public Health website (www.fph.org.uk) or the UK Public Health Careers website (www.phorcast.org.uk).

A PERSONAL PERSPECTIVE ON THE UK SPECIALIST TRAINING PROGRAMME

Amy Potter, Specialty Registrar in Public Health (ST4/4th year of training)

A Specialty Registrar (StR) in Public Health is part of the national training programme to develop Public Health Consultants. In the UK the body that oversees training and professional standards is the Faculty of Public Health (FPH) (1).[1]

Public Health StRs come from a variety of medical and non-medical backgrounds, but once in training, there is no distinction between the two groups in terms of training curriculum, opportunities and assessment. Training is usually over five years, although previous experience may be taken into account, and covers knowledge and practice in the three key domains of public health practice: health protection, health improvement, and health and social care services. StRs are supported through training by a training programme director and by educational supervisors in each placement.

The training

During the first of three phases of training, StRs typically complete an academic course such as a Master of Public Health covering core topics such as epidemiology and statistics, disease causation and prevention, social policy, health economics and organisation of healthcare. Phase 1 usually lasts about two years, and also includes some time working in a local public health department[2] and for a local Health Protection Unit providing the public health response to infectious diseases in the UK.

The end of Phase 1 is marked by starting Health Protection 'On Call' work and successful completion of the first of two FPH exams: the Part A 'knowledge' exam. This is followed six to nine months later by the Part B 'demonstration' exam where the focus is more on translating knowledge into practice (2). After passing both exams, StRs officially become members of the FPH (MFPH).

Meanwhile, underpinning all this is a range of competencies that have to be met throughout training in order to demonstrate a good grasp and experience of different aspects of public health practice, from surveillance and assessment of population heath; the ability to collect intelligence and assess evidence and to work collaboratively to develop appropriate policies and strategies, as well as developing an ability to understand and use different leadership styles to achieve change (3).

The move into the final phase of training comprises completion of the required competencies. This usually happens about eighteen months before training finishes with the award of CCT (Certificate of Completion of Training).[3] In this final phase, and depending on which competencies are still outstanding, StRs have access to a broad range of opportunities, including placements in academia, with charitable sector organisations working on public health issues or advocacy, or at national level, e.g. with the National Institute for Health and Care Excellence (NICE) or government departments such as the Department of Health.

Registration

At the end of training, Public Health Consultants must be registered to practise, either with the General Medical Council (4), or with the UK Public Health Register (5) if from a background other than medicine. Dentists have a separate, but comparable training programme, leading to specialist registration in dental public health with the General Dental Council.

My route into specialist training

As with many of my colleagues, I came to public health in a roundabout route, taking a while to realise that it was 'public health' that drew together for me a seemingly disparate range of interests: effective management of health services, tackling inequalities in access to care, and the upstream determinants of health such as housing, education and community cohesion.

As a science undergraduate, I specialised in pathology, and while studying the histology and immunology of infection, began to think about the genetic and social factors that determine why some people are more at risk of becoming ill than others. This led me to a Master's (M.Sc.) in Control of Infectious Diseases at the London

School of Hygiene & Tropical Medicine (LSHTM), focusing on Low and Middle Income Countries (LMIC), which enabled me to explore some of these social aspects of epidemiology, health and healthcare.

I subsequently worked with an organisation called THET (6) which aimed to increase the capacity of health workers in LMICs through training and support provided by long-term links with health institutions in the UK. As a result, I became interested in the role of effective health management and health systems in improving health, and applied to the two-year NHS Graduate Management Scheme (7), wanting to gain practical skills and experience in organisational management and leadership. Through this scheme and after graduating from it, I worked in primary and secondary care NHS organisations in London while undertaking an M.Sc. in Healthcare Leadership and Management. I had the opportunity to see real changes to services that patients received, including markedly reduced waiting times and shorter post-operative lengths of stay, but after a few years I became frustrated that I spent most of my time 'fire-fighting' rather than strategically improving services, and was also discouraged by the often fractious relationship between clinicians and managers, despite what I felt was our shared vision to improve services for patients. I took a break from the NHS, working with a relief and development agency called Tearfund (8) in post-conflict Liberia, West Africa, managing health and community development projects.

Returning to the UK with fresh perspective, and wanting to work in a more strategic role, I changed tack from health management to public health and found myself in a remarkably similar job in East London to the one I had been doing in West Africa (only with fewer mosquitoes), working on strategies to improve people's lifestyle choices. I managed a local health trainer service,[4] and worked in partnership with primary care, the local authority, the voluntary sector and the public in order to increase immunisation uptake, improve care for chronic conditions, address wider determinants of health and reduce inequalities, and discovered that I loved it.

Through colleagues, I heard about the public health training scheme, and the pieces of my career to date suddenly fell into place as I realised that 'public health' gave cohesion to what had seemed diverse topics: strategic action and partnership to tackle the upstream determinants of health and wellbeing, and ensuring that well-organised health and social services are available that meet need, particularly of the most vulnerable in society.

Not coming from a medical background, I had not realised that I could apply for specialist public health training until I was working in a public health department with StRs on placement. Although some aspects of being part of a 'medical' specialty are still a bit bemusing (What's an ST1?[5] How do I get a CCT? When on call for the Health Protection Unit, what do I do when people assume I must be a doctor and start reeling off long lists of medical acronyms?), one of the most stimulating things about working in public health is the variety of backgrounds and interests that we as a discipline have, and experiencing how we can complement each other's skills and experience.

Public Health StRs are a core part of the public health workforce, often carrying out essential projects that other public health staff do not have the capacity to do. Specialist public health training offers a fantastic opportunity to work in varied areas and organisations, and to get the opportunity to try different career options out for size. To illustrate, the following is a sample of the work I have been able to do:

- I completed a large-scale health needs assessment for local Community Health Services (CHS) and, through disseminating the findings, observed that front-line district nurses and health visitors gain a different perspective on their role in organising health and social care services around the patient, that managers were enabled to use their activity data to check that their services are meeting anticipated local need, and saw my work used as a basis for commissioning services in a different way.
- As part of a national working group to develop new public health guidelines for dealing with typhoid, I reviewed the evidence base for the existing guidelines and made recommendations, which has led to a significant change in the public health management of typhoid cases throughout the UK, ensuring that resources are targeted more effectively.
- More recently, I have been working as a researcher within the International Centre for Eye Health at LSHTM. This has enabled me to explore a career in academia, to teach on the M.Sc. in Public Health, develop and evaluate training materials, and teach international ophthalmology students about health systems on a summer short course. This experience highlighted a passion for communicating ideas and supporting others to learn, and has also been important for giving me confidence about my own knowledge and ability. I aim to maintain links with research and teaching in the future.

Roles and career opportunities

Public Health Consultants look at the 'bigger picture' in tackling poor health and its causes, and I am of the opinion that if you try hard enough, you can define almost anything as 'public health' if it has an impact on health and wellbeing. As such, there are roles and opportunities for Public Health Consultants in a multitude of settings, both in the UK and abroad (9). The following are just a few, but the world really is your oyster when it comes to a meaningful career in improving population health and reducing inequalities:

- working with locally elected councillors and local authorities to analyse the role of employment, social isolation and other wider determinants of health in the local population, and implementing evidence-based programmes to integrate services;
- supporting the new Clinical Commissioning Groups to help GP leaders to map their population's health needs (including those who never attend their GP surgery), understand need, demand and supply, and to commission appropriate services;
- working in a hospital with external health and social care partners, including the voluntary sector, to integrate health and social care, to improve early diagnosis and appropriate discharge, making sure that services are joined up for those with multiple chronic conditions or social care needs;

- leading the development of evidence-based policy and programmes for national or international charities, government bodies or think tanks working in national or global health;
- undertaking research to provide a robust evidence base for public health advocacy, policy and practice nationally or internationally, and teaching the next generation of public health experts.

Despite the current uncertainty around what the public health function locally and nationally within the UK will look like over the coming years, change always creates opportunity and there will always be a need for experienced public health practitioners, whatever the organisational structures look like.

At a recent training event, I was discussing with a group of StRs what gave us joy about working in public health, and once we got started, we found it hard to stop. There is an enormous sense of pride in the profession, that we are part of a long chain of historical figures who have made a significant impact on population health, from Edwin Chadwick[6] to Michael Marmot.[7] Many talked about the fact that public health as a discipline enabled us to match both personal values and skill set or expertise, giving personal satisfaction as well as intellectual challenge. Effective working in public health is impossible without collaboration; getting things done with and through others, and the diversity in roles, backgrounds, topic areas, actors and organisations involved in public health practice are a real stimulant.

Skills needed as a Specialty Registrar in Public Health

Effective public health practice requires a careful balance between generalism and specialism: not forgetting the big picture and the upstream causes of poor health and health inequalities, but also having the ability to look in enough detail at the evidence, using analytical skills to figure out the root causes and appraise the evidence for interventions. It requires a love of enquiry and investigation, of detective work to think about why the situation is as it is, combined with creativity and vision to imagine how it might look in the future.

Much of the epidemiology, statistics and other building blocks that form the foundation of work as a public health specialist can be taught through the M.Sc., but to really enjoy public health and use your skills to make an impact requires an interest in the 'but why?' and the 'so what?' questions, a desire not only to understand the data but to go a step further to think about what it *means*, bringing the evidence base to life and making it practical. To lead the change required to improve population health needs an ability to use data to influence decisions, to enjoy communicating ideas with passion and vision, and to take time to build relationships, to work through others and be content not necessarily to get the credit but to see progress towards longer term goals, and to seize opportunities to move things forward.

The public health training scheme is an ideal time to learn how different organisations work, to experiment with different leadership styles and ways of working as an individual or in teams, to practise negotiating and influencing skills, and to work with people from a variety of different professional and organisational backgrounds. It requires adaptability and a willingness to get involved; there are always interesting projects but you may have to be bold and search them out.

How to get started if you are interested in training to be a Public Health Consultant

If you are interested in specialising in public health, there are a number of standard resources available which give you the nuts and bolts of what a career in public health involves, details of the qualifications required and annual recruitment process and an overview of training (1, 10–11). Each Deanery website will give more details of each area's training programme, as well as giving key contacts of training programme directors[8] and often registrar reps[9] too. There are also resources that registrars have put together to help individuals and organisations recognise and understand the value of the work that StRs do on a daily basis – for instance, the 'Meet Reg' project from the Yorkshire and the Humber Deanery: www.yorksandhumberdeanery.nhs.uk/public_health/meet_reg/index.html.

To get an idea of how public health is organised in the UK as well as current public health priorities, you need to:

- familiarise yourself with key government policies such as White Papers and related policy documents that discuss organisational changes, structures and who is responsible for delivering which aspects of public health;
- read journal articles and learn to critically appraise the study design and conclusions;
- follow the vocal #publichealth crowd on Twitter to see what they are talking about (a great way to keep up with the latest policy developments) and even join in with a discussion on the Public Health Twitter Journal Club #PHTwitJC;
- develop a habit of reading the newspaper with a public health hat on, looking for stories about cancer drugs, obesity, vaccination or funding decisions for health services, taking note of the strength of evidence cited and the experts quoted, often public health specialists;
- organise to spend time in a local public health department, especially if you are straight from a hospital-based medical background, and/or volunteer with a local voluntary sector organisation to gain perspective on some of the social and political determinants of health and wellbeing, and challenges to individual and population behaviour change.

Notes

1   Numbers in brackets refer to Website references below.
2   Previously these would have been within Primary Care Trusts, but following the Health and Social Care Act in 2012, future Phase 1 placements are likely to be in local authorities or Clinical Commissioning Groups.

3 A CCT confirms that a specialty registrar has completed an approved training programme and is eligible for entry on to the General Medical Council (GMC) Specialist Register or the UK Public Health Register – a requirement for NHS consultant practice.
4 Local people trained to improve health in their community.
5 A specialty registrar in year 1 of specialist training.
6 A social reformer in England in the 1800s, noted for his work to reform the Poor Laws, link poor living conditions to risk of disease and improve municipal sanitation.
7 A Professor of Epidemiology and Public Health in London, who has been involved in seminal public health research and policy during his career, including the Whitehall Studies of risk factors for cardiovascular disease in British civil servants, and the more recent Marmot Review into health inequalities in England in 2010: Fair Society, Healthy Lives. Sir Michael also chaired the WHO Commission on Social Determinants of Health: Closing the Gap in a Generation, which reported in 2008.
8 Training Programme Directors, or TPDs, manage the specialist training programme in an area, coordinating and communicating between registrars, educational supervisors, the postgraduate dean and the FPH.
9 Registrar reps are chosen by their peers to represent the voice of registrars to their Deanery and on national committees such as the Specialty Registrars Committee (SRC), a formal subgroup of the FPH Education Committee.

Website references

(1) Faculty of Public Health. Public Health Careers: Specialise in the 'bigger picture'. Available online at: www.fph.org.uk/public_health_careers. Accessed 24 January 2013.
(2) Faculty of Public Health. FPH Exams Available online at: www.fph.org.uk/exams. Accessed 20 January 2013.
(3) Faculty of Public Health. Public Health Specialty Training Curriculum 2010. Available online at: www.fph.org.uk/uploads/2010MASTERPHCurriculum0610b.pdf. Accessed 20 April 2014.
(4) GMC. General Medical Council. Available online at: www.gmc-uk.org/index.asp. Accessed 24 January 2013.
(5) UKPHR. UK Public Health Register. Available online at: www.publichealthregister. org.uk. Accessed 24 January 2013.
(6) THET. The Tropical Health and Education Trust website. Available online at: www.thet.org. Accessed January 2013.
(7) NHS Leadership Academy. NHS Graduate Management Scheme website. Available online at: www.nhsgraduates.co.uk. Accessed 20 January 2013.
(8) Tearfund. Tearfund website. Available online at: www.tearfund.org. Accessed 30 January 2013.
(9) Faculty of Public Health. Being a public health consultant. Available online at: www. fph.org.uk/being_a_public_health_consultant. Accessed 24 January 2013.
(10) The Gold Guide: A Reference Guide for Postgraduate Specialty Training in the UK. 3rd edn. 2009. Available online at: http://specialtytraining.hee.nhs.uk/wp-content/uploads/sites/475/2013/10/Gold-Guide-2010.pdf. Accessed 20 April 2014.
(11) Faculty of Public Health. Recruitment into the Public Health Training Programme. 2013. Available online at: www.fph.org.uk/recruitment. Accessed 26 January 2013.

14 Personal and professional development in public health

Em Rahman

Introduction

New knowledge is forever appearing in the field of public health, so practitioners have to be prepared to work throughout their working lives to ensure that they remain up to date. A particular tenet of public health practice is the application of the 'evidence base' to all that we do, and it is therefore incumbent upon all of us to keep up to speed with emerging evidence and, indeed, to contribute to the published evidence by participating in research whenever feasible, and by writing articles for publication in peer reviewed journals.

Public health entails, therefore, commitment to life-long learning and application of the best available evidence to all that we do. The commonly used term for this ongoing development is continuing professional development (CPD). While on a formal training course or at university or college, this development is the main feature of our professional life. The trick is to ensure that it remains central well after we have completed the requirements of training for a particular role and throughout life whether or not we aspire to progress in our career by further job changes or promotion. To comply with best practice, every public health practitioner should engage in an annual cycle of CPD, tailored to meet their personal needs as described in their own personal development plan (PDP), with progress monitored at their annual professional appraisal. While all this probably sounds very bureaucratic and time-consuming, having the opportunity to organise one's own development and having regular opportunities for feedback to check to see if the plan is realistic and meeting our needs, is actually surprisingly liberating.

One reason for including in this part of the book the description below of approaches to personal development is that it demonstrates the importance of self-directed learning and development. As we have read, in some areas of public health practice, there is as yet little by way of formal training or career development routes, so 'do it yourself' is the norm. In addition, you can begin your own development to become a public health practitioner through adopting a habit of CPD and PDP, in order to take your career in the direction of public health; you will then be as well prepared as possible when you decide to apply for your first public health role.

A LIFE IN PUBLIC HEALTH WORKFORCE DEVELOPMENT

Em Rahman, Public Health Workforce Development, Wessex Deanery

There are many different approaches to developing essential new skills at all stages of your life and your career. The *Oxford Dictionary* defines *development* as: 'A specified state of growth or advancement; the process of developing or being developed'.

Why is development important?

Development is about growth and advancement that is enabled by a process or structure that allows the individual to progress along a pathway, therefore providing development for an individual. When any individual begins to explore their career plans or personal development plans, it is important to start by asking the question 'Where do you see yourself in five years?' By asking this question individuals can begin to unpick what it is they need to do now in order to achieve their future goal. Aspiring to progress and develop in any career is important and needs to be harnessed by the organisation and line managers. If you are not yet employed and are considering a career in public health, then it may be useful to seek the support or advice of a careers adviser – at school, university or other place of study, or independently – or make contact with your local public health team. If you are in employment, then personal development should be an integral part of your appraisal and supervision meetings.

Assessing what development you might need

Using the UK Public Health Skills and Careers framework (Skills for Health, 2008) (accessed through www.phorcast.org.uk) provides a helpful point of reference of the skills and knowledge required to progress up the different levels in public health. There is also a self-assessment checklist on the website. By exploring where you are currently and what additional skills and knowledge are required for you to progress can help inform what type of development you may need to undertake to achieve your goals – for example, it may be a qualification or course that may be required if you need to develop your knowledge.

Another approach you can take is to explore the different roles that exist within public health[1], which will help you understand the context and landscape of the public health workforce and also the types of roles that might interest you now and in the future. This is a useful exercise as you can look at what is needed for specific roles and then work to develop your skills to meet the requirements.

What is the scope of professional and personal development?

Development can take place in a variety of methods from 'learning in the role' to much more formal academic courses. What will be important is for you to be able to keep a record of all your personal development achievements so that you are able to demonstrate the skills and knowledge that you have gained. The range of development that individuals may normally encounter is as follows.

Project work/work-based learning

A large proportion of any individual's development will take place in the workplace as they work in their roles. This can be where individuals have gained a skill or developed their knowledge by being involved in a project or piece of work.

Accredited courses

These will be courses that have some sort of qualification or accreditation process attached to them. These may be a university degree in Public Health or an accredited short training course on behaviour change, for instance. Keeping a record of not only the qualification certificate but the learning outcomes/objectives of the course will help you to demonstrate (and remind you) what you learned on the course.

Non-accredited courses

These types of courses are usually internal courses to an organisation and will usually include mandatory training such as Health and Safety, Safeguarding and Fire Safety, etc. The mandatory courses may be different for different people depending on their role and responsibility. There may also be opportunities for individuals to access other non-mandatory training that their organisation's Learning and Development team may deliver, such as project management or train the trainer, etc. Linking in with your organisation's Learning and Development team will be useful in understanding what is on offer for you and your colleagues.

Conferences

Attending conferences can provide an update for individuals on the topic that the conference is focusing on – for example, if it is a general public health conference or a specific conference on obesity. Some conferences will highlight that they are CPD (continuing professional development) certified, which means that attendance to that conference can be counted towards an individual's CPD.

Continuing professional development (CPD)

Continuing professional development should be an integral part of any role and become normal practice for anyone wishing to develop and progress. In public health you will find the majority of individuals keep a CPD portfolio, which will include their evidence for demonstrating their continuing professional development, and this is particularly important if individuals are required to evidence their CPD in order to maintain registration or likewise will be useful for individuals who are working towards professional registration.

Reflective practice

Using reflective practice models as a way of learning and developing can be very powerful. If there is an incident or issue that an individual has gained a great deal from, then it may be useful to write a short reflective piece as evidence of development but also to embed the learning gained. A simple approach to reflective practice is the following:

- **What?** What happened? Report the facts and events of an experience, objectively.
- **So what?** What was your experience? How was it different from what you expected?
- **Now what?** What is the future impact? What will you do differently? What's the learning that can be shared?

How to approach development

If you want to develop a career in public health, then approaching your own development in a proactive way will be a good idea. It will also be good to work on your development plan with someone (e.g. your line manager or a careers adviser or mentor). This is good practice for everyone, in public health or anywhere.

There are three broad steps to creating your development plan. These are:

1   Where do you want to be in five years, say?
- What role do you want to be doing?
- Which domains of public health do you want to be working in?
- What do you not want to be doing?
- What level of responsibility do you see yourself having?
- How much do you see yourself earning?

2   What do you need to do in the next two years?
- What knowledge do I need?
- What skills do I need?
- What knowledge and skills do I already have?
- Is what I want to achieve in five years realistic?

- Who can I access for support?
- What is available to me now?
- What do you need to do/can you do in the short term?
- What do you need to do/can you do in the long term?

3   Produce a personal development action plan (often called a PDP).
- Do you need to work towards a qualification or complete a course?
- Are you keeping a CPD portfolio?
- Do you need to work towards professional registration?
- Have you spoken to anyone doing the role/at the level that you want to be in five years?
- Have you highlighted this as part of your appraisal?

By exploring the above points and questions you will begin to see your personal development plan coming together; remember to keep this plan live and review regularly to see what you have achieved, what you have not achieved and why not, and what you need to achieve moving forward.

How to approach courses before you start to ensure you get the best out of them

When starting any course, whether it is a degree or a short course, it is important that you link this back to your development plan in order to maximise on the learning and development you will gain. Before starting any course you should look at how this course will help your development in both the short and long term. For example, you may need to do a course or some training to support you in your current role. However, there may also be courses you do that will support your development in the long run but not necessarily in your current role/work.

In order to gain the most out of your learning, it will be useful to understand more about you and the learner you are, whether your preference is to learn by doing or learn by thinking, etc. This self-awareness can help you understand how you approach a course and how you continue on the course. For example, you may find a course that has a mixture of group work and role play more effective if your preference is to learn by doing.

For courses that require some sort of assessment or assignment, it may be helpful to focus the assignments to work you are already doing in order to get the most out of it. This way you are able to apply the learning from the course to your own practice as well as complete your course and your work.

How to seek funding support

There are a range of funding and support opportunities that may be available, although these are not consistent across the UK or over time. If you need financial support to complete a course and are in employment, the first port of call should be your line manager. If the course has been identified as part of your role or your development, then your employing organisation should be finding resources to support you in this. Therefore, it is crucial that your personal development plan is signed off and agreed by your line manager. If that is not possible, you may need to look out for education bursaries that may be being provided locally, regionally or nationally. It will be important for you to understand that you may not get the support you need in order to develop straight away, but try not to get disheartened, and, unless you can pay for the course yourself, you may just need to keep on raising it with your line manager or, where appropriate, human resources adviser as a development need for you.

Good luck!

Note

1   Use the vignettes on the UK Public Health Careers Website, www.phorcast.org.uk. Available online at: www.skillsforhealth.org.uk/search/public%20health/?ordering= newest&searchphrase=all. Accessed 10 November 2013.

Reference

Skills for Health, *UK Public Health and Skills Career Framework*, 2008. Available online at: www.skillsforhealth.org.uk/search/public%20health/?ordering=newest&searchphrase =all. Accessed 10 November 2013.

Part 5

How to proceed from here
Fiona Sim and Jenny Wright

Introduction

The book so far has set out a range of perspectives on public health careers. It has shown the huge variety or careers and potential opportunities, and how to access them, whatever your specific interest and existing skill set.

We wanted to be sure that no one is under the illusion that there is one simple and straightforward pathway to a career in public health, and we think that has been achieved. On the contrary, you have read how broad the discipline of public health is and how varied are the careers on offer. We hope you will also have found out what motivates public health practitioners and why they believe this is such a rewarding career. The enthusiasm of public health people is contagious. As one contributor pointed out: 'We [public health practitioners at all levels] are very willing to share our experiences!'

For many careers in public health the requirements in terms of your initial qualifications, from school or university, are not set out rigidly and, indeed, the public health community is well known for its appreciation of people with diverse skills and background experience when they come along with a commitment to improve the health of the population. While a generation ago, to become a public health specialist you had first to qualify as a doctor and practise clinical medicine for at least three years before entering public health training, now you can be eligible to specialise in public health with any good first degree and enough work experience and maturity of attitude to demonstrate your understanding of, and passion for, population health.

To practise public health in roles other than consultant, the entry requirements are even more flexible. You will have read that to be a health trainer, for example, you need to be able to communicate with ordinary people and want to work with your community to help people to improve their health and wellbeing. Once appointed to a training position, tailored training will then be provided to ensure that you can offer suitable advice and be effective in the role.

To specialise in health intelligence, you will need to be comfortable around numbers and be able to conduct mathematical analysis and interpretation, while to work in health promotion, communication skills and an understanding of how people learn, behave and make decisions are paramount.

To be a public health practitioner, therefore, you can start with aptitude and interest in a very wide variety of things and bring them to the discipline. One thing is sure, if you bring your skills, we can help you to use them to benefit the health and wellbeing of the population.

Attitudes are important

First, you need to have a belief in lifelong learning: the field of public health and the evidence of what works is changing very rapidly, so it won't do to take up a job and think you will be competent to do it for the whole of your career. Even if the job remains largely unchanged (which is unlikely), the skills and knowledge you need will continue to evolve and it will be essential to update your skills continuously throughout your career. This has been well described by Em Rahman in Chapter 14.

Next, it is crucial that you can work with long timescales. There are very few times when there is instant gratification in public health practice, with perhaps the main exceptions being teaching, when you can hope to see your students succeed relatively soon after teaching them, and the control of outbreaks of communicable disease, where a bigger problem is averted by your team's prompt action. In much of public health practice, real change in population health status takes years or decades to emerge, so we learn to work with interim goals to ensure we are on track towards the main objective. As a consequence of the time it takes to achieve meaningful change, the population for whom you work will not thank you for changing their lives, and there are no grateful patients or satisfied customers. So if you need instant gratification, public health is not for you; if you can cope with the long haul, it is.

Rewards in public health

To dispel another myth – in case it is out there somewhere – people do not become public health practitioners in order to become millionaires. There is little scope for materialism in public health practice. The values you will have noticed in reading the chapters of this book demonstrate a passion for making the world a fairer place, reducing preventable inequalities, for improving the health of communities, especially those in greatest need, the poor and those whose voice is not otherwise heard.

But not everyone is driven by great financial reward and public health practitioners are actually paid quite well in comparison with many other disciplines. The public health practitioner is perhaps more likely to be driven by seeing the results of their hard work, whether this is about getting members of a local inner city community in urban England with poor levels of physical activity to embark on a healthy physical exercise regime – which will in time lead to reductions in premature deaths from heart disease – or about introducing a vaccine campaign in rural India – which will lead to fewer deaths from polio – the job satisfaction is clear: your efforts will have made a difference to the lives of real people in real communities. And since public health practitioners almost always work as part of a multiprofessional team, you will have the added pleasure of working with others and learning from your team mates, as they will learn from you.

A note about terminology

Throughout the book, there are references to public health practitioners being 'medical' or 'non-medical'. This merits some explanation. Until the late 1990s, specialist practice in public health (by 'consultants') was confined to those who had completed specialist training in public health medicine, and the training programmes were open only to medical graduates. When the training programmes opened to people from backgrounds other than medicine in the early 2000s, they were described in the accurate, but rather negative term 'non-medical' practitioners, trainees, specialists or consultants. In the continued absence of a suitable alternative term, we have continued to use the term 'non-medical'. In reality in 2014, it makes little difference to the range of jobs available to public health practitioners whether or not you have a medical qualification, but for doctors, public health has always opened up a whole host of career opportunities not available in typical clinical practice, and continues to do so. And since the quality of the public health workforce is enriched by the inclusion of practitioners from so many different core disciplines, we hope that people from a medical background will long continue to be part of the multidisciplinary public health family.

If you want to be a public health practitioner, what do you do next?

Now you are ready to get going. As you will have seen, there are many routes into public health work but do not let this put you off. Some public health careers have clear pathways, others do not have such formal routes or qualification. Many people move into public health from other careers or jobs. Use the information on the UK Public Health Careers website to help you with some of the detail (www.phorcast. org.uk). It will also signpost you to a whole host of other useful websites that will help you decide which direction is best for you.

There are some simple steps to begin with:

- Explore the different roles, functions and settings.
- Decide what interests you most.
- Decide which appeals most either as an end point or at a stage on your career path.
- Consider the skills and knowledge you bring and those additional ones you might need for specific roles or careers (self-assess on PHORCaST).
- Talk to people, look at PHORCaST examples, consider volunteering or internships to get some initial experience.
- Look at whether you need any formal qualifications, courses and where and how you may attain them.

Do remember: nearly everyone who works in public health is enthusiastic about their chosen career, so do not be shy about making contact if you are interested in a career in public health. As well as considering making an enquiry to your local public health team, you can contact one or more of the public health organisations mentioned in the book and listed in Appendix 2.

A small warning: there are always exceptions to the enthusiasm that we have described. For example, the public health system is reorganised often by successive governments; public health practitioners, perhaps especially those in leadership positions, tend to tire of reapplying for similar roles in newly reconfigured organisations and so you may come across some of this soon after a period of transition as a new system beds in, the most recent system reform having happened in 2013. In addition, a change of government will always bring with it some changes in public policy that may be more or less sympathetic to the overarching goals of public health practice. This can affect the morale of the public health workforce or individuals within it if they feel that their professional priorities and passion are no longer well aligned with those of government. Most changes, however, will present the public health practitioner with new opportunities.

Please do make use of the goodwill that you will discover by showing interest in a career in public health. Most people do not know what public health is, so you are already well ahead of the game and your enquiry will sound highly motivated and intelligent by the time you get to this point in the book.

More about PHORCaST, the Public Health Online Resource for Careers, Skills and Training

Several contributors have referred to PHORCaST throughout the book, so we were keen to have an up-to-date understanding about its future. Here is an update from Jonathan Bardill, Public Health Careers Website Manager, Health Education East Midlands:

> PHORCaST is the first 'one-stop shop' for UK-wide information on careers and development in public health, and health and wellbeing. It provides general information on public health, details about the wide variety of roles available, the skills and qualifications required to get into those roles, real-life career stories, advice on personal development, information on accessing relevant education and training opportunities, and selected news, events and documents related to public health.
>
> From the autumn of 2014, a new Health Education England website for health careers information will be available, and will incorporate the material that currently appears on PHORCaST, NHS Careers and Medical Careers in a new information architecture. This is a major change, which will result in a much improved health careers web service, providing users with a much broader perspective on the available careers in health. Visitors to PHORCaST will be automatically redirected to the new site [www.phorcast.org.uk].

Concluding remarks from the editors

This takes us to the point at which we hope you have enough information to help you to explore further if your interest has been sparked by any of the material in the foregoing chapters. If you have been inspired to consider a career in public health, we wish you all the best in your chosen field and look forward to meeting you or hearing from you in years to come. Perhaps it is worth reminding readers that, as several of the contributors to this book have described, public health is commonly a field that is discovered or rediscovered in mid-career; this often leads to a second career, so if you are unsure at this stage that public health is for you, you might want to return to this book in a while and see if you are inspired to join the global community of public health practitioners at a later date.

Finally, good luck. If at some time you do choose a career in the diverse and everchanging world of public health, you will never be bored and you will not be disappointed.

Appendix 1

About the contributors
to this book

Fiona Sim. I studied Medicine at University College London (UCL), when public health was a tiny part of the course. Then I trained to be a GP. I soon became aware of my interest in prevention, which was incompatible with my partners' smoking in their consulting rooms! When I spotted an advertisement in the *British Medical Journal* for specialist training in what was then called Community Medicine, which included the opportunity to apply to do a Master's course at the London School of Hygiene & Tropical Medicine, I was seduced. I was appointed to the training programme despite a conspicuous lack of knowledge, but maybe the genuine interest shone through. After training, which I completed when I was thirty, I had no game plan and went on to hold a series of senior roles in public health, NHS management, academia and the civil service, including Director of Public Health, Trust Medical Director, Associate Dean of Postgraduate Medicine, Coordinator of London's Teaching Public Health Network and Head of Public Health Development for England, where, among other responsibilities, I led the establishment of voluntary regulation of public health specialists. A strong theme throughout my career, mostly through voluntary positions and research, has been teaching, and training and professional development. I have been Director of Training for the Faculty of Public Health, Registrar of the UK Public Health Register and a trainer in both public health and general practice.

One of the great strengths of public health knowledge and skills is their transferability, so a whole world of job opportunities opens for those of us who find the skills and the imagination to use them creatively. Boredom is not an option. Personally, I never really mastered the so-called work–life balance and had many years of guilty motherhood when I tried too hard to get it right and probably missed many of my children's early achievements, but they tolerated their errant parent and never showed any resentment of my career. It has taken a long time to get here, but now I have achieved a satisfying and varied portfolio of work: I am a part-time GP in a socially deprived area, a Clinical Director of my local Clinical Commissioning Group and a Senior Clinical Adviser to NHS England Area Team. In my spare time, I continue to indulge my passion for building public health capacity: I am Chair of the Royal Society for Public Health and joint Editor-in-Chief of the international peer reviewed journal, *Public Health*, and have honorary academic positions at University of Bedfordshire and the London School of Hygiene and Tropical Medicine.

I am passionate about building capacity across all sectors to deliver better population health and reduce inequalities – hence this book.

Jenny Wright. When I graduated with a degree in Modern History I had no clear idea of what I wanted to do beyond being interested in social sciences and trying to make the world a better place. I qualified as a social worker, then moved into social science and health services research, where I completed a Master's degree in Philosophy. This led me to several health and social care service planning posts. My last planning post was at regional health level and in a public health department. When regional health authorities were disbanded, the public health department I was in established itself as an independent business unit within the health service, undertaking contract work for a range of organisations, including the Department of Health, local health service organisations, charities and local authorities. It was during this time that I developed a passion for public health development and furthering the interests of the public health workforce in all its guises. I was fortunate enough to undertake national work involved with the setting up of the UK Public Health Register processes, developing the retrospective portfolio assessment framework. I was able to qualify myself as a specialist. I later worked with Skills for Health, on behalf of the Department of Health (DH), to develop the UK Public Health Skills and Career (competence) framework. It was while I was overseeing for the DH the Teaching Public Health Networks programme that I met Fiona. Before I retired, I led the team developing and running the UK Public Health Careers website for the UK Departments of Health. I am now undertaking a part-time doctorate, researching women public health doctors.

Jenny Amery trained as a public health physician. Early in her career she worked in Latin America for nine years, focusing on the health of poor women and children, and community development. Dr Amery led DFID's work on health in Latin America, later became regional adviser for South Asia and then DFID Head of Profession Health and Education.

Diane Bell trained and worked as a hospital physician, then in public health medicine. She has been a visiting Fellow at the King's Fund, Director of Strategy and Planning for NHS Milton Keynes and a 2010–2011 Commonwealth Fund Harkness Fellow in the USA. She is currently Director of Strategy and System Redesign at NHS Bedfordshire Clinical Commissioning Group.

Katie Cole was inspired to pursue a career in public health while studying Medicine at the University of Birmingham. She obtained a B.Sc. in International Health from University College London and a Master of Public Health (MPH) from the London School of Hygiene & Tropical Medicine, and has since been training to be a Consultant in Public Health.

Surindar Dhesi is a freelance chartered environmental health practitioner, writing her Ph.D. on Health and Wellbeing Boards, health inequalities and environmental health in 2014. She holds a B.Sc. (Hons) in Environmental Health, an M.Sc. in Public Health and a NEBOSH Diploma. She is a founder member of the UK Environmental Health Research Network.

Clare Ebberson started as a management trainee in local government, gaining diverse experience in housing, parks and democratic services. Later she worked in local government policy teams and joint health needs assessment between health and local government. Now a specialty registrar, Clare has an M.Phil. in Public Health and a Postgraduate Diploma in Public Service Leadership and Management.

Claire Everett began her working life in sports development until an increasing interest in nutrition led her to study B.Sc. Human Nutrition and M.Sc. Food and Nutrition Policy. She has worked across all sectors in roles related to environmental health, public health, catering and education, and is a visiting university lecturer.

Frances Fairman. A passion for getting evidence into practice, combined with an M.Sc. in Healthcare Policy and Management, and a commitment to ongoing learning, enabled Frances Fairman's career to progress from NHS administrator to Clinical Effectiveness Manager with NHS Central Southern Commissioning Support Unit, and with it, the satisfaction of contributing to improved population health and access to NHS care.

Ian Gray. After taking A-levels in 1969, Ian Gray studied for four years to obtain his Public Health Inspectors Diploma in 1973. After a long career in local government, he became a specialist at the Health Development Agency in 2000 and then Principal Policy Officer at the Chartered Institute of Environmental Health, leading on public health and health protection.

Rebecca Hams. Now a specialty Registrar in Public Health, Rebecca Hams was previously involved in a collaborative project, bringing together NHS organisations, local authorities, and public- and private-sector organisations to improve the health of a county. Her previous research is related to childhood obesity. She has an M.Phil. in Public Health and an M.Sc. in Paediatric Exercise Physiology.

Alison Hill is Public Health England's Deputy Chief Knowledge Officer. She has over twenty-five years' public health experience within the NHS, and has particular expertise in health evidence and intelligence to improve health and reduce health inequalities. Her previous jobs included Managing Director of Solutions for Public Health and Director of Public Health in Buckinghamshire.

Helen Hogan is a Clinical Lecturer in Public Health and M.Sc. Course Director. She is qualified in Medicine and holds an M.Sc. in Public Health. She joined the London School of Hygiene & Tropical Medicine in 2006, following completion of public health training in the NHS. Prior to this she was a GP. Her research interests are in patient safety in NHS hospitals and she has recently completed a Ph.D. in this area.

Manuelle Hurwitz is a Senior Adviser for the International Planned Parenthood Federation (IPPF). Prior to joining IPPF, Manuelle worked as Research Officer for the University of Oxford. Manuelle has a BA in Social Anthropology and an M.Sc. in Medical Demography. She has a special interest in working towards social justice and equity of access in health.

Muireann Kelly is a first-year doctoral student in the Faculty of Health and Social Care at London South Bank University. Her research examines the potential role of nurses as exemplars for healthy living. She holds a BA in Psychology from National University of Ireland, Galway, and an M.Sc. in Public Health from the London School of Hygiene & Tropical Medicine.

Paul Lincoln has worked in public health at local, national and international levels in the public and third sector for thirty-two years, and been an educational adviser, teacher and researcher. He is currently Chief Executive of the UK Health Forum, which focuses on the primary prevention of linked avoidable non-communicable diseases. He is a member of many government, NICE and other scientific expert public health advisory groups.

Sue Lloyd is a registered public health specialist. She is director of a successful public health consultancy, Nutrition and Wellbeing Ltd. She is also chair of the UK Public Health Register Registration Panel, where she supports the development of both public health specialists and practitioners in the UK.

Martin McKee is Professor of European Public Health at the London School of Hygiene & Tropical Medicine where he created the European Centre on Health of Societies in Transition (ECOHOST), a WHO Collaborating Centre, and is also Research Director of the European Observatory on Health Systems and Policies.

Richard Parish was Chief Executive of the Royal Society for Public Health until July 2013, having previously held senior NHS and academic appointments. A consultant to WHO for over twenty years, he is now a member of the Public Health England Board. Richard chairs the Pharmacy and Public Health Forum for England and is a UKPHR Board Member.

Anita Parkin worked in academic statistics and health economics after a Maths degree, then in the NHS in various information, performance and public health intelligence roles. She has worked in the Department of Public Health, appointed jointly to two different local authorities, one in the South East and one in the North of England. Her Ph.D. was in deprivation and health.

Amy Potter is currently a Health Adviser for the UK Department for International Development (DFID). She studied Natural Sciences (Pathology) as an undergraduate and has Master's degrees in Control of Infectious Diseases (2004) and Healthcare Leadership and Management (2008). She is in the last phase of training to qualify as a registered Public Health Consultant, having completed the Faculty of Public Health professional examinations.

Em Rahman (European Health Promotion Practitioner, registered with IUHPE) has worked in public health since 2001 and currently leads public health workforce development for Wessex region, supporting the training, education and development of public health practitioners and wider public health workforces. Em is passionate about supporting individuals to develop their public health careers and recognises the need to develop public health career pathways at all levels.

Mala Rao is Professor of International Health, University of East London, and Honorary Consultant, Public Health England. Her public health career has spanned practice, policy, research and teaching in the NHS, and has taken her from the local to national and global arenas.

Duncan Selbie is Chief Executive, Public Health England. From 2007 to 2012 he was Chief Executive of Brighton and Sussex University Hospitals and from 2003 to 2007 Director General of Programmes and Performance for the NHS, and subsequently was the first Director General of Commissioning. Previously he was Chief Executive of South East London Strategic Health Authority and South West London and St George's Mental Health NHS Trust. He joined the NHS on 1 January 1980.

Martin Seymour gained extensive experience in local government before moving into public health, initially as a health improvement specialist. He previously worked on a national programme supporting local government to address health inequalities. Now a specialty registrar, he completed an M.Sc. in Public Health, writing on collaborative advantage for health improvement from strategic partnership working.

Mohit Sharma trained as a surgeon in India and then worked in the NHS. Within public health training he worked in a range of placements with national organisations and with local authorities. He is now working with Public Health England, teaches medical students in Oxford, and is a member of a research ethics committee.

Peter Sheridan was a GP before training in public health. He was Director of Public Health in Enfield before joining the Health Protection Agency. He is self-employed and works with local authorities and supports medical performance for Public Health England. He is Registrar of the Faculty of Public Health.

Manpreet Singh is currently a Senior Consultant on health and development for Dalberg Global Development Advisors in Nairobi. His previous experience spans a wide range in global health, from clinical medicine, to social entrepreneurship, to research and teaching. Manpreet has a Master of Public Health degree. His advice is: be persistent!

Lorna Willcox qualified as an Environmental Health Officer in 1992 following a B.Sc. in Environmental Health at Greenwich University and practical training at Woking Borough Council. She worked in food and safety enforcement in Northampton and

Kettering, and joined Public Health England in 2013 as a Health Protection Practitioner. Her article on Safety at Paintball Games appeared in 1994 and she took part in filming the BBC's *Food Inspectors* (2011).

Jane Wills is Professor of Health Promotion at London South Bank University. She teaches on the M.Sc. Public Health and Health Promotion course, writes textbooks on the practice of health promotion, and carries out research and evaluations funded locally and nationally. Her early career was in educational research and school teaching.

Jan Yates has a background in teaching and moved into public health, completing specialist training in 2008. She worked for three years as a Director of Public Health and more recently her main focus has been on assuring the quality of public health screening programmes at regional and national level, while maintaining a strong interest in training and development.

Appendix 2
Useful professional organisations for public health

Chartered Institute of Environmental Health (CIEH) sets standards, accredits courses and awards qualifications for environmental health practitioners in England, Wales and Northern Ireland. Available online at: www.cieh.org

Faculty of Public Health (FPH) is a faculty of the Royal College of Physicians, which acts as the UK standard setting body for public health specialists from any disciplinary background. Available online at: www.fph.org.uk

General Dental Council (GDC) is a regulatory body for all dentists and public health dentists in the UK. Available online at: www.gdc-uk.org

General Medical Council (GMC) is a regulatory body for all doctors working in the UK. Available online at: www.gmc-uk.org

General Pharmaceutical Council (GPhC) is a regulatory body for pharmacists and pharmacy technicians in the UK. Available online at: www.pharmacyregulation.org

Health and Care Professions Council (HCPC) is a regulatory body for several health and social care professions in the UK. Available online at: www.hpc-uk.org

International Union for Health Promotion and Education (IUHPE) is an independent professional association of individuals and organisations committed to improving population health and wellbeing through education, community action and healthy public policy. Available online at: www.iuhpe.org

NHS Education Scotland is a special health board responsible for developing and delivering education and training for those who work in NHS Scotland. Available online at: www.nes.scot.nhs.uk

Nursing and Midwifery Council (NMC) is a regulatory body for nurses, including public health nurses, in the UK. Available online at: www.nmc-uk.org

Public Health Agency, Northern Ireland is responsible for public health improvement, health protection, health and social care commissioning, advice and research and development. Available online at: www.publichealth.hscni.net

Public Health England (PHE) is a civil service national agency for public health in England. Available online at: www.gov.uk/government/organisations/public-health-england

Public Health Wales is the national public health service for Wales. Available online at: www.publichealthwales.wales.nhs.uk

The Royal Environmental Health Institute of Scotland (REHIS) is the regulator for environmental health officers in Scotland. Available online at: www.rehis.com

Royal Society for Public Health (RSPH) is an independent charity to promote and protect human health and wellbeing; an international membership organisation open to anyone interested in public health, including student membership; and provides policy advocacy, qualifications and training. Available online at: www.rsph.org.uk and www.publichealth.hscni.net

UK Public Health Register (UKPHR) is an independent regulatory body for public health specialists and practitioners. Available online at: www.publichealthregister.org.uk

Index

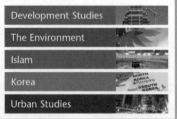